TO *Kale*

AND

Back

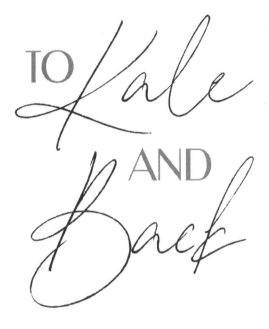

TO Kale AND Back

DITCH THE RULES
AND LEARN TO THRIVE
IN FOOD, FITNESS, AND LIFE

DIANA MATUSZAK

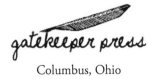

gatekeeper press
Columbus, Ohio

To Kale and Back: Ditch the Rules and Learn to
Thrive in Food, Fitness, and Life

Published by Gatekeeper Press
2167 Stringtown Rd, Suite 109
Columbus, OH 43123-2989
www.GatekeeperPress.com

Cover photo by Katie Rae Bode

ISBN (paperback): 9781642376425
eISBN: 9781642376432

Printed in the United States of America

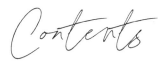

Contents

Introduction

"Shout out to all of the girls out there trying to love themselves in a world that is constantly telling them not to."

—Anonymous

I AM A CERTIFIED holistic health coach, and I hate kale. It's true. Is that even possible? And get this—I also can't stand avocados that aren't in guacamole form. Am I even #healthy? Yes. Yes, I am. Here's the deal though, friends. I haven't always accepted my non-poster-child of health-like self. I want to share my journey to *true* health and wellness with you in hopes to help you find your most balanced healthy lifestyle too (with or without kale), and build the confidence to create your dream life.

Circa five years ago, I was like, "Self-love? What on earth does that mean? Be so desperately self-centered and self-righteous, and always make decisions based on your own good? Sounds like a selfish witch with a capital B if you ask me."

And then the whole "you are enough" preachers. I would

have said, "Damn straight I'm enough. I am a smart, driven, cute-haired, going to run the world Beyoncé-type of girl. Okay? Glad we got that settled."

Alright, alright. Let's back up here. I definitely would think and tell myself all of those things repeatedly. I'd tell myself that I had my shizit together and I was going down the right path, but it's as if there were two very conflicting versions of me. On the one hand, I was convinced I actually was enough, but I also told myself I wouldn't attract my dream man until I had a flat stomach. That I wouldn't be my "best self" until I achieved what everyone else viewed as a dream body. I thought, "I'll finally be living my best life when the last roll on my stomach goes away. I am such a healthy person for only eating salad today. I'm bound to get the perfect body and finally feel complete."

I only wish I'd taken the time to see what everyone meant by true self-love and worthiness, then I might have seen the poop with a capital S that I was about to put myself through just to get that body, and what I thought was "the life."

What I'm here to tell you is that self-love is not selfish. Loving yourself at every stage only helps you to achieve your goals faster. Treating yourself with more respect helps you serve others better. You are enough as you are, and are able to have every damn dream you've ever dreamt up. You are worthy of a love so strong that it allows you to feel at peace and happy every single day.

I remember reading things like this back then and thinking, "Well, okay, cool, but how do you get to that place of knowing? Easy for you to say, you have the dream body and life." Much easier said than done, but that's why I'm here. That's why I'm writing this book—to show you how to do that. To show you how to push past the toxicity of society, how to find TRUE health and wellness without restriction or rigidity, how to feel confident in your own skin every darn day and create the life of your dreams. And I don't mean any of that lightly. It's available to you, friend. Time to start living it. Spoiler alert . . . it doesn't happen when you find all of those things, but you bet your buttons I'll show you where to find it.

Sadly, the core of these beliefs (self-love, worthiness, and enough-ness) for many lies in weight and appearance. Society places so much emphasis on appearance that we begin to be blinded by it. Here's the secret, though. You CAN have that dream body. You can and you will, but not without a healthy amount of self-love and appreciation along the way. The end all be all is not just the body, it's the confidence, relationship, job, energy, and level of happiness we *think* the body will bring us.

Trust me. I eventually found what I thought was my "dream body" before I found my way to true health. I was so focused on looking better, going further, doing more, "it's not enough yet," "it's not perfect yet," that I had absolutely no idea I'd actually reached that thinner body I wanted from the beginning. I was so consumed with not being enough and trying to be "better" that I couldn't even see the thinner version of me staring back in the mirror. I was missing quite a few key pieces. I'm going to tell you those key pieces so that you, friend, can slide right past all of my mistakes and get right to the end goal of confidence, happiness, and your dream life without the excess struggle.

Let's start at the beginning, shall we?

I'll never forget my third grade teacher, let's call her Mrs.

W. I loved her, mostly because she always complimented my hairstyle. I'm pretty sure I had a different hairstyle with cute little hair ties and bows every single day, thanks to Mom who was and is the supermom of all moms. You know what I'm talking about—those pigtails where you put hair ties all the way down the remaining hair so they're like bubble braids? Yep, mom was definitely Supermom.

"Alright, on the next section, I want each of you to write down your weight on the second line," said Mrs. W. Looking back, I'm not quite sure what the lesson was getting at. Were we learning compare and contrast concepts? Maybe something math oriented? All I remember is what happened next, because it has stuck with me like it was yesterday for the past sixteen years.

"Corey, may I use you as an example for the class? What did you write down?" asked Mrs. W.

"Seventy-six pounds," said Corey.

"Wow, really? Hmm, well, I guess you *are* pretty tall, aren't you? Okay," Mrs. W. responded.

My eight-year-old mind froze. "What? He's just tall? Corey is much taller than me, but I wrote down eighty-two? Is that bad? I'm not tall. Why is my number higher than his? What does that mean? Am I ugly? Do people not like me?" I thought.

The rest of the morning I felt self-conscious.

Am I fat?

Do my friends tease me behind my back?

Do they make fun of me and I don't notice?

Until this point, I was just your average eight-year-old with exceptionally fabulous hair. I had noticed that other kids had different body shapes, most being smaller than mine. I hadn't had the belief that one was better than the other, or one was good and one was bad, one gets teased the other doesn't. Not until then.

Ring ring ring! The bell chimed, indicating it was finally time for recess. All of the other third graders and I smiled and ran as fast as we could outside to the playground. Finally! Time for the monkey bars! Looking back, I'm not sure how I have healthy skin on my hands as an adult. Blisters always covered my hands from those darn monkey bars. As per usual, my girlfriends and I ran to the play set. No matter how blistered our hands were, we never missed a recess period on the monkey bars. We'd race, see who could jump to the farthest bar, and make obstacle courses by skipping certain bars. We were basically eight-year-old professional monkey barers (not a word, but you catch my drift). Jumping into our usual routine, we played all of our silly games just as we did every other day, but this day was different. That day will remain in the back of my mind for the rest of my life.

When Kristina jumped off the monkey bars and bent over to sit down, I noticed something I'd never noticed before.

When she bent over, I could see the trail of her spine sticking out, the up and down outline of her vertebrae visible as her shirt inched up over her belt.

Kristina was a very pretty eight-year-old girl. She had a lot of friends, she was smart, the teachers liked her, many of the boys had crushes on her, and she was a great friend. She was also much smaller than me, like a lot of the other girls.

I looked around the playground and noticed the rest of my friends' bodies. Almost every one of their spines stuck out when they bent over too.

"My spine doesn't stick out when I bend over," I thought.

"Why doesn't my spine stick out?"

"Why aren't I normal and like all of the other girls?"

"Is that why my number was higher than Corey's?"

"Why did Mrs. W say it was because he's tall?"

"Does that mean I'm fat?"

From what I remember, that day sort of came and went, but it brought an awareness I'd never had in my eight short years of life.

That was my first exposure to body image. My first exposure to fat versus thin, good versus bad, pretty versus ugly, big versus small. I don't blame Mrs. W. one bit. I don't think she had any idea what impact writing down our weights would have on a young mind, nor do I think she intended to do any harm. That is the scary part though—messages like that occur every single day. We often have no discretion over which messages young children hear and which ones they don't, or how they interpret them, especially when we're not there to supervise.

Holy heck. Reason number five hundred million two hundred seventy-five that I am writing this book. Did you know that, "Approximately 91% of women are unhappy with their bodies and resort to dieting [over balanced lifestyle changes] to achieve their ideal body shape." And, "More than one-third of people who admit to 'normal dieting,' will merge into pathological dieting. Roughly a quarter of those will suffer from a partial or full-on eating-disorder."[1]

Sweet baby Jesus, this needs to change. It starts with you

---

1   "11 facts about body image," Do Something, (https://www.dosomething.org/us/facts/11-facts-about-body-image).

and me. I'm guiding you to freedom from food, cultivating self-love and confidence so that you too can be a role model for true health and wellbeing right along with me, so that our children do not have to grow up in this environment that we currently have. Are you with me? Give me an amen, sister! Jersey shore fist pump and say "heck yes we're doing this." We're changing the world, my friend. Great, glad we've got that covered. Back to the story!

I would eventually be diagnosed with Insulin Resistance Syndrome. High blood pressure, high blood sugar, high cholesterol—you name it, I had it at ten years old. But remember, I had Supermom and Superdad! No fear to be had. With incredible support, we did everything we could to change my lifestyle at age ten and turn my diabetic-fate around. I became very athletic, playing every sport out there, which brought me into high school as a healthy teenager. And then came college.

Freshman fifteen? I think we should call it the "freshman start to eat like a typical seven-year-old and gain weight faster than you can say 'party at the neighbor's.'" But I guess "freshman fifteen" is easier to say, isn't it? The freshman fifteen was all too real for me. Despite how many times I'd said I'd *never* be that girl. I loved working out, which I did nearly every day. Not only that, but through my past lifestyle changes, I truly liked eating healthier foods, too. It just so happened that those occasional college tendencies to choose chicken tenders and french fries over well-balanced meals grew more and more frequent than it once had. How did that turn out?

Well, ladies and gents, it turns out that raspberry Smirnoff mixed with orange Fanta in your best friend's boyfriend's dorm room every weekend isn't exactly fit-body friendly. What?! Say it ain't so! What about the fruity pebbles in my frozen yogurt in the dining hall? EXCUSE ME?! Those aren't fit-body friendly either?! LORD ALMIGHTY WHY DID YOU HAVE TO PUT CALORIES AND SUGAR IN MY PRECIOUS ICE CREAM!?

Ugh. Life is just mean sometimes, isn't it?

All jokes aside. How did food go from being something that gives us life and creates energy to live our best days—a privilege to be provided with high-quality nourishing foods—to the idea that food is something that either makes us fat or makes us skinny? That we must manipulate it in a very detailed and specific way if we want to achieve a certain body? That there is a list of good foods and a list of bad? If you ever want to achieve that goal-body, that you better swear over the holy bible you'll never touch the list of no's? When did this even get put into the realm of "healthy" either? Google healthy weight loss and I promise you the top results will include restrictive diets, manipulation of food, and how to find a quick-fix result. Maybe that's why it's more common to attempt to destroy your body (unknowingly at the time, of course) than to just create a sustainable healthy lifestyle.

If you can't tell by now, I am an advocate for *sustainable healthy* lifestyles and have been since the beginning of my career as a health and wellness coach. Maybe you're wondering how I even became a health and wellness coach. So glad you asked!

I began my career in the corporate world. As you'll find out later, I went through many struggles in college. Toward the end of college and after copious amounts of difficult inner-work, self-improvement, and self-love, I developed a strong affinity for nutrition and wellness and wondered if I should've majored in that instead. But I was good at accounting, really good. As in, I received awards in college for my success and my friends asked me to do their homework just so they could pass, that good. So merging my love for business as well as health and wellness became the next best option. To be honest, I didn't hate it. *Cue all of the nerdy accounting jokes.* Don't worry, I've heard them all.

In my first career, I was a licensed CPA (certified public accountant) for a large public accounting firm, but I always held the vision that one day I would work for a wellness company. Whether it be fitness or nutrition, going into wellness was my end goal. I was inspired to do this, of course, because of my story and my desire to help others. I could feel God's tug on my heart to go the wellness direction. I opened my heart to God's inspiration, and one day I found the Health Coach Institute. I enrolled almost immediately for the certification program and felt a sense of ease that this was truly my calling. Plenty of late-night and ungodly-early study sessions later, as well as juggling my passion with my job, I became a certified Health and Life Coach. Feeling God's reassurance, I enrolled further and am now a certified *Transformation* Expert. More about this later, but I said bye-bye to my cushy, secure, high-paying corporate job to follow my heart and make an impact on the world.

Since the beginning of my career as a health and wellness coach, I *always* tailor programs to clients' lifestyles. For those who want to lose weight, we don't focus on what we're taking away, but rather add as much of the good as we can. I encourage them not to say "no" to all of the things they love, like happy hours or Sunday pancakes with the kiddos, if they don't want to. And you know what? They have healthier cravings. They lose weight. They keep it off. And for all of my clients, whether weight loss is a goal or not, they stop going through guilt from food decisions. They find a love for their body, and they ultimately begin to live their dream lives. It's that simple, and it should be that simple for you too.

When I look back at the course of my life, from all of my health concerns, to helping so many amazing women find their best health and life, I find such wonder and awe in the Big Guy upstairs —God, the universe, Big Man/Goddess upstairs, whoever you choose, insert their name here—and His magnificent plan for us..

I know this to be true: for a very important reason, God put me through these experiences:

1. Being unhealthily overweight

2. Being unaware of what makes a food nutritious or not

3. Losing weight by meticulously manipulating and constantly thinking about food

4. Being afraid of something as nutritious as an apple because of the belief that the sugar will bring back all of the fat I'd lost

5. Uncontrollable bingeing.

Quite the wide spectrum, eh? Sometimes difficult times lead to beautiful destinies. This is mine—experiencing every side of the spectrum of unhealthy so that I can make a change in this world. I will guide you to your healthiest relationship with food and body, your most balanced healthy lifestyle, so you can create ultimate confidence in your own skin, and the develop the tenacity to create a passionate and fulfilling life. This is my promise to you.

Clearly, somewhere along the way, we got everything mixed up. We began to believe that other people know better than us and that we need to outsource our nutrition to someone else just to lose fifteen pounds. If we don't, it will take way too long, and we won't get the results we want. We even started to believe that just understanding food and nutrition and a balanced healthy lifestyle isn't enough. We began to believe that learning what a gift food is and how the different macro and micronutrients help you create the body, mindset, and confidence of your dreams just isn't enough, either.

Another spoiler alert. It is enough. It's everything actually.

I've tried just about every single wrong way to create what I thought was a healthy body. I began with seeing my health and worth as how many muscles I could see or how many abs I had. And just a little side note, the Big Guy upstairs blessed me with the body type that I early-on perceived and labeled as "apple shaped" and carried with me throughout my life. Not sure what that is? Well, you see, I always seemed to lose fat in my big toe before my stomach. I know, tragic. For as long as I can remember, this is how I perceived my body. Legs are okay, but that darn stomach. It was never good enough, flat enough, tight enough.

The fact that I was using my belly as a determinant for whether or not I was successful is INSANE IN THE MEMBRANE. A recipe for catastrophe. Wow, this may actually turn into a poem at some point. But I digress.

Honestly, I had the legs of a runway model and a booty like J. Lo, but my blinded eyes only saw that roll on my stomach. I had become one of those people without a weight problem, complaining about my weight. I was more self-conscious with the body so many girls dreamed to have than the one I had when I was fifteen pounds heavier. See, this is the power of the words you use with yourself. Would you talk to your three-year-old daughter in the same manner as you do yourself? A friend? Your sister? Your mother?

See, friends, I've been on this journey a heck of a long time. Changing these perceptions of myself, beginning to see my beauty in the mirror before my perceived imperfections, and actually talking to myself as if I'm on the same team instead of the enemy has taken me years of incredibly hard work. It probably took so long because of the years I'd spent getting really good at hating it. Ending the habit of looking to see if I'd become Susie Six Pack in literally every mirror I passed was a hard one to quit.

I had it all wrong by focusing on the outward appearances over my mind, body, and soul. For a long time, I didn't see emotional and mental health as important along with the physical appearance. We have this stigma in our world where we're all just hush hush about mental health. Like if you feel you need therapy, there's something "wrong" with you. Or if you're depressed or in a really negative place with yourself, you're "messed up." NO MY FRIENDS, DAS WRONG. Nope. Incorrect. Asking for help is a sign of strength. Working to better your mental state is one of the healthiest things you can do. It helps you create your best life.

But here's the thing, friend. I have a different point of

view than many body positivity advocates out there. I don't think there's anything wrong with working to better yourself, or become the most fit, strongest version of yourself, even if that means losing or gaining weight. Why? The point of being the healthiest version of you is to live the highest quality of life possible. So having the energy to play with the little rascals when they come home from school, move hundreds of boxes up and down the stairs of your new home you got to purchase because God surprised you with twins, try amazing new things like hiking to the top of Sky Pond in Colorado, or something as simple as walk up a flight of stairs without getting winded is part of living a high-quality of life. I am all about beauty at every size. We are all beautiful, absolutely no exceptions. What I do also stand for is empowering each other to be the *healthiest* version of ourselves as well.

If you have a goal of trading your slurpee for a smoothie to become a healthier version of you by losing some extra weight, more power to you. You radiate happiness and confidence when you feel your absolute best every single day. Acquiring this sort of confidence opens new doors in life you never knew existed, because accomplishing something as gratifying as shaping your healthiest, strongest, fittest, or most confident body plants a seed of courage and determination within that not many other things can plant. When we approach weight loss/gain, fitness, strength, stamina, or creating the body of your dreams with the mindset that we are striving to live life to the fullest, to be as healthy as possible so we can fulfill God's plan for us, to create the energy and confidence needed to pursue the scariest of all scary yet exciting opportunities in life, to be the best mom we can, to be the best wife, sister, or daughter possible, to be a light to the world and a source of happiness and abundance, then by golly friend, it is good. But we must also know that we can have and be all of these things without killing ourselves for the flat stomach.

It's funny how it works, but once you actually realize and *believe* this, the body naturally follows. I know, I know, I can feel you through the pages. You're annoyed. "Okay, cool. I've read that a million times, but I don't believe it and I don't feel it." I know, I've been there too. Many times actually. By the end of this book, you'll believe it, you'll feel it, and you'll be creating the health, body, mindset, and confidence of your dreams.

I say I've been there because let me tell you, I was stubborn. I stayed in that place of standing in my own way for years. And now, my dear, I know the truth. Life is too short to be uncomfortable in your own skin. Too short to hold back from doing things you've always dreamt of because you live in a world of self-doubt, lack of self-confidence, or being held back because of your weight or body image.

And this, so far, is only my story, but we all have a story. This speaks to all of us at some degree.

It speaks to all of the mamas out there, trying to figure out if it's safe to do squats while holding your infant as a weight because there's just not enough time in the day. Or pureeing all of the veggies into a poop-looking soupy substance that you're actually going to make your baby eat because you are wholeheartedly invested in your child's nutrition, but not in your own. Child first, mommy last? Maybe, but mommy needs some TLC too.

It speaks to all of the boss babes climbing the corporate

ladder and blasting through the glass ceiling. Oh, the meeting is getting pushed into lunch time? Lovely. I just adore finally being able to eat a meal again when I feel like I'm as hungry as a black bear getting ready for hibernation, eating absolutely everything in sight. Oh, and Debbie made brownies again? Can't make her feel bad, better have one for dessert. Might as well feed me coffee through an IV this afternoon. Does it have to be that way? No. Is that normal? Absolutely. I've lived the corporate life, I've seen the way it works. You can and you will break that glass ceiling if that's what you so desire. But you will also do it so much faster while living your absolute healthiest and happiest life too, sans the pressure of co-workers and uncontrollable lunch meetings. There is a trick for everything.

Truly, it is so much more than weight, what you look like, and how many muscles you can see. It affects absolutely every other area of life. When I work with my coaching clients, we look at it from every single angle. I teach them how, according to the experts at Health Coach Institute and the model I have used in my coaching practice, quality of life is divided into these key parts:

- Health
- Relationships
- Career & Money
- Spirituality

The quality of our health from the point of view of mind, body, and soul is affected by every single one of these.

They say that the way you do one thing is the way you do everything. If health is out of whack, chances are something else is too.

What does this mean? It's incredibly difficult to reach our full potential, create the life of our dreams, and be truly happy if all areas are not at their best. So we need to approach it from every single angle. In the rest of this book, I am going to lay it all out for you. We'll hit every aspect of trouble and debunk all of the myths.

We'll look at childhood and how the way you're brought up greatly affects weight, body image, and sense of happiness and wellbeing in adulthood. Obviously, making it difficult to change if we don't approach it from this angle.

We'll look at relationships to keep you from ending up with dumb-butts and dip-poops with a capital S so that you can find your soulmate and Prince Charming, your knight in shining armor. But hopefully not literally wearing armor because that would be weird. While we're on this topic, my experience is as a woman in romantic relationships and mostly female friendships, but whenever I reference going out and scooping up your fabulous life partner, insert your side of the story there. Are you a man looking for your lady friend? Or a gal looking for your fabulous gal pal for life? Or a man looking for your Prince Charming? Apply it to your life, you do you friend!

We'll look at friendships. The Regina Georges of the world and how to stand up for yourself when you just want the Serena and Blair sort of relationship.

We'll look at the gym and exercise and see if it's worth sweating your tush off at those scorching hot-as-the-devil's-lair yoga classes. I mean, hot yoga.

We'll look at nutrition, how to hate kale and still be a healthy human being with a body you're incredibly confident in. Diving deep into why Ben, Jerry, and Mr. Orville Redenbacher are your favorite Friday night dates.

And finally, career, the future, and success, because if travelling the world and saving all of the kitties and puppies in an animal resort is your life's dream, then do it, sister. Or maybe going into marketing sounds safe and secure but psychology is your favorite subject. Well, buy that couch tomorrow because you can be darn good at anything you want to be. Your passion is your purpose. I'll show you how to find your purpose and passion, and how to start living your dream successful life right now.

You can see that my point of view is one that says treating our bodies with real, high-quality foods is oh-so-important, along with saying goodbye to food guilt, and I'll show you exactly how to do that, but it's not everything. Healing our minds to think positive thoughts, finding happiness in every day, and seeing what we *love* about ourselves rather than what we hate is a major part of being truly healthy, happy, and confident. And by doing so, eating healthy nutritious foods will be what we actually *want* to do because doing anything less would just not make sense. Lastly, when we find our own personal healthy lifestyle, we will become so magnetically happy, so confident, and so purpose-driven that living anything but our absolute best life will be unacceptable and absurd. Have the courage to pursue your dreams. If you're not happy, you have the power to change it.

But remember, I am not a doctor, I am not a psychiatrist. My professional training would have me asking you to please love yourself enough to seek help if your struggles interfere with your performance at work or school, family life, social life, the ability to function in everyday tasks, or are life-threatening.

My hope is that this book inspires humans around the world to ditch the toxic self-hate at any level and cultivate self-love so strong that it creates a ripple effect. So that one day, our children never experience the load of toxic messages we experience today. Soon, we will be a population of joyful, peaceful, fearless, money-making, passionate, full-of-love human beings. I would add more adjectives but I'm getting confused with that sentence myself. We'll be happy and healthy AF (as fudge), okay?

It's all available to you. Yes, every single one of you no matter what, no exceptions. First, you have to believe it; second, you have to decide what you want; and third, you don't stop until you're living it.

I'm here to show you exactly how to do that, to show you every single mistake I've made so that you can either jump ship if you're experiencing that too or miss it by a million miles so that you can start living your healthiest, *best life ever*. Today.

You may feel really compelled to just skip over the "step by step" part of each chapter—the one where you have to get up and grab a pen. I know, I'm sorry. Yes, I'm going to make you do it. This is where the transformation begins and the progress starts to take place. Trust me, you're going to want to do the steps in this book!

Now raise your champagne, dirty martini, IPA beer, or sparkling water with lime in a champagne glass and cheers to that, friend.

CHAPTER 1

*Go home Edna,
you're drunk.*

"That sounds like a terrible idea . . . what time?"

—All of us at some point in life.

PEOPLE EVERYWHERE ARE doing juice cleanses, detoxes, and fad diets like it's nobody's business. In reality, it's just full of a whole lot of society bull poop. Do they make enemas for that? Gross. Ew. Too far. My bad.

But seriously, if that big-old thing we call society wasn't so royally F-ed up, things like juice cleanses would be seen for what they really are, which is a big, fat *Suzie lost her marbles again because celery juice just doesn't cut it for a week.* While we're at it, let's rename society, shall we? I feel seriously gross and dirty when I say that word because it's so full of bull poop I can't stand it. We shall call her Edna. Shut up, Edna. Edna, sit down.

Yesterday, I was standing in line at Publix for the third time this week because I needed raspberries on top of my smoothie to make it perfect and all of my raspberries were moldy. Raspberries, can you please stay fresh for at least forty-eight hours? You're more high maintenance than the Kardashians.

Anywho, the man in front of me decided he was special and took thirty-two things into the express lane, so there I waited. Unsurprisingly, I saw the cover of one of those trash magazines, as Supermom likes to call them, in the checkout line with the front-page title reading "Lose twenty pounds in two weeks with this proven soup method!" I opened the pages to this *lovely* article because I just had to see what nonsense they were talking about this time. What they failed to mention are the fabulous side effects of gaining back thirty pounds in the third week and becoming the Wicked Witch of the West in the process.

A couple of months ago, I got engaged (finally, go babe! Love you!), so of course I've purchased literally every over-priced bridal magazine in my line of vision for the past six months. Yes, I did buy way too many before we were even engaged. Don't act like you've never opened one. Don't lie to me! This is a judgment-free zone, okay?

An overwhelming majority of them have *at least* one article about "why you *need* to be doing only this workout," "try this diet for the last three months of your engagement," yada yada yada. Make it stop. BUT! I did read one recently in *Brides Magazine* about using health and fitness as a stress reliever, something to make the planning a tad less stressful and help keep you feeling your very best. There is hope!

Hold on, let's rewind back to the Kardashians for a

second. Y'all have a fabulous show. Seriously. But if I see one more headline about how all of you baby-makers lost the baby weight seconds after your child was born and bounced back just a week later with a tighter-than-pre-baby body, I WILL HAVE A SERIOUS COW.

Alright, can you see the trend I'm showing you right now? Edna is full of extremely biased and misused pieces of information that we just love to dramatize. Edna is a drama queen. Edna does have a good side to her and I have hope that she is growing, but that girl needs some serious Jesus. The majority of Edna's messages are enema-worthy, causing people to do horrible things like cabbage soup cleanses, juice detoxes, and hate themselves, continuously finding fault more often than loving themselves. Honestly, some aren't even that extreme, so they might *sound* like Edna strengthening her good-girl muscle, but she's not. It's an act. She's a filthy lying Regina George of the bunch most of the time.

I give you, "Do [insert diet trend here] and lose the last ten pounds fast!" There are so many diets out there like keto, paleo, Atkins, and more. I want to be clear though too. You are not "bad" for trying these things. In fact, sometimes they *can* be beneficial. For example, *my* version of balance (stay tuned) includes a little clean-up of my diet,meaning the foods I eat, for about a week every time I feel I need it, because I physically feel my best on whole foods, even though I also love chips and fries.

But Edna doesn't like to highlight the instances when these are beneficial, outside of strict weight-loss regimens and for the sake of a quick fix. She also very rarely focuses on methods that make you an all-around better human being (mind, body, and soul), which finding health and wellness truly does. She misses a major point! When you use these more regimented diets for some appropriate reasons, great—give it a shot:

1. Medicinal reasons
2. Experimental purposes, such as to find the root of a foodborne issue
3. Figuring out where certain symptoms are coming from (under appropriate guidance)
4. Treating a foodborne illness

Of course, this isn't an exhaustive list, but if you're using a diet solely for the purpose of losing thirty pounds before that trip to Mexico where your friend invited McDreamy pants and you have to impress him regardless of how much you hate your life in the process, let me stop you right there.

Have you checked into *why* you're only eating the foods on the "allowed" list? Do you understand where the benefits are coming from, or how to implement it in a balanced way? Are you more focused on the flat-stomach-result that is promised?

Oh, but Sir Flex-A-Lot swears by it!

It's the same old story. I'm pretty experienced myself when it comes to getting so excited about the possible weight loss that I've given it the old college try. Many times.

During the middle of spring semester—well into the first year of raspberry Smirnoff mixed with Orange Fanta, fruity pebbles in my froyo, and twenty pounds later—I decided

I needed a turnaround. I signed up for the university's half-marathon and felt readier than ever to get rid of those rolls that appeared out of nowhere (or did they though? Hmm . . .). Four months later and hundreds of miles in, I still wasn't seeing the results I was hoping for. Summer came, and I continued my efforts down the yellow brick road to the Emerald City, also known as, "let's just get back to the weight I was before." At the time, even though I didn't see my desired results, I thought I must be doing something right. An ex-boyfriend, Nick, came running back—the one who had broken up with me senior year of high school and left me in a pool of my own tears for a solid month.

Hmm, he's still attracted to me. I must be on the right path.

Let me just remind you that up until about the end of spring semester of my freshman year of college when I'd decided to focus solely on weight loss, I was the life of the party. For example, heading into the decision-making process of figuring out which dorm party or house party we need to be at that night, I had only one question.

"Is there going to be dancing?" I would ask.

"Probably not, dancing is probably at the baseball house," a girlfriend would say.

"We should probably head to the baseball house then," I would reply in my skinny jeans and heals, raspberry Smirnoff and Orange Fanta in hand. I would already have two tallies on my hand—we were clever back then, marking our hands with a sharpie for each drink we'd had that night. Wake up feeling like you got hit by a bus? Check the tallies on your hand. Whoops.

Until weight loss became my sole focus, I had been very

confident in myself. I didn't have abs or the "perfect" body, but I felt good. I carried myself confidently. Cute boy there? We didn't leave until I talked to him. Cute top showing a little midriff? I wore it. Tight dress with an open back? I bought it.

During this confident period, one of my best friends and I were sitting in Spanish class one day and our professor (she was so cool, I totally would have hung out with her at a dorm party), asked us to discuss in Spanish the qualities of our perfect man or partner to practice our new vocabulary.

"Diana, how would you and Lydia describe your ideal man or partner?" she asked.

We replied "alto, oscuro, guapo, y un atleta," or "tall, dark, handsome and an athlete" for my non-Spanish speakers out there.

Behind us, Sara muffled under her breath, "jersey-chaser."

To which I replied, "We don't chase jerseys, the jerseys chase us."

Stunned at my quick reply but also a little proud, we laughed.

See? Even on the path down the freshman fifteen, my confidence was stronger than ever.

But by the end of spring semester and into the summer following my freshman year, I began to feel disconnected from my confident self. It was as if I could suddenly feel all of the weight I'd gained just sitting on my body, tearing away at my own sense of my beauty. I would no longer wear tight dresses. I felt self-conscious getting into a bathing suit, my sense of self-love and confidence became a distant memory. I looked in the mirror and all I could see were flaws. How could I let myself get this far? I thought. "How could I lose myself like this? If I try to talk to that boy, maybe he won't give me the time of day anymore."

At that point, I didn't care about abs yet. I didn't want to look like a fitness model. I just wanted to feel good and confident again. By the time summer came, I'd decided I was making changes. I'd clean up my nutrition and start to exercise a bit more intentionally. After a few months of eating healthier but just not getting the results I'd hoped for, I began to do some "research." This is where Edna so rudely invited herself to my party.

Turning to my new obsession, Pinterest, I became preoccupied with looking at the "health and fitness" page. What did I find? Articles upon articles titled something like "Eat These Foods and See Results Fast," "If You Want to Lose the Last Ten Pounds, Stop Eating This," "Why You Should Never Eat Bananas Again," and "How Alcohol is Ruining Fat Loss Progress." They might as well have just said that bread is the devil's soul-food and if you eat anything on the "no" list it's worse than robbing a bank.

Believe it or not, I'm actually a pretty smart person. I graduated high school as Valedictorian and received a five-year degree in four years with an extensive minor, but apparently my smarty pants brain cells did not catch this one. That darn Edna, sneaky b**ch. Well, that, and I was now desperate for my dream body. I wanted nothing more than to look like that fitness model.

I thought to myself, "Well, it's all over the internet, it must be true."

So I did what the gurus said. It began slow. I thought of some things as healthy, some not, but did them anyway. I stopped eating cereal bars for breakfast, added a few more veggies to my lunch. Then it escalated. I stopped drinking alcohol altogether. I downloaded a calorie tracking app, entered my goals, and the weight finally began to shed. My confidence, on the other hand, depended on the number on the scale. Not yet where I wanted it to be, I still didn't feel good enough or pretty enough. My confidence remained at rock bottom.

Before I could even comprehend what was happening, my obsession went further and further. I never ate more than what the app said to do by even a calorie. In fact, I started to think it was better to eat even less than the app recommended. I never understood the principles behind how many calories I should be eating, I only focused on reducing my intake like the app told me to, often taking it even further.

"1,200 calories to lose weight? 1,100 must be better," I thought.

The results became addicting, in the same way that researching and trying out the "best" ways to a flat stomach became addicting. None of those articles I read discussed balance or having french fries every now and then. They never mentioned nourishing your emotional health with self-love and appreciation. Certainly none of them said it was okay to not track my intake on the calorie tracking app I'd made my lifeline. No days off, right?

Some rational part of me knew this was wrong—that it didn't have to be this extreme. I knew that I shouldn't have to cut things out entirely, but the emotional part of me so desperately wanted to see myself as pretty again. I just wanted to feel good like I once had, and I wanted it right away. The emotional part of me muted the rational part of me. Key word? Emotions. The emotions that were at the center of my beliefs. My beliefs of not being enough, never going to be pretty enough, funny enough, likeable enough—all caused me to go straight to extremes without registering what I was doing to my body and mind.

It's easier for Edna to be the life of the party with extremes rather than give balanced lifestyle messages. Therefore, I did not believe I could have the results I desired fast enough without the extreme methods Edna loved to highlight. I never allowed myself to believe that maybe Edna was wrong in her extreme teaching. Ten pounds became twelve, twelve became fifteen, fifteen became twenty-five.

It's funny (not so funny) how it happens. In my pre-college body, I didn't have abs. I wasn't "fitspo," but I radiated confidence anyway. The weight began to pile on, twenty pounds later I no longer felt that confidence inside of me. I lost the weight. Then I lost a lot more. It became an addiction. As my sense of beauty and worth became validated by the number on the scale my confidence plummeted further than I'd ever experienced before. All of the weight I'd gained was gone, and plenty more. But my obsession with getting smaller, having the Edna-proclaimed "perfect body," and constantly needing to look better put up a wall where confidence and self-love just couldn't get over anymore. I needed balance, but had no idea what that even meant. I lost connection with my friends. I lost myself. Before I knew it, I was alone, afraid of many foods, including alcohol, and the only fruit I would eat was blueberries because that's all that the gurus said was okay.

The scarier part than the fear and the aloneness? I was blinded to the fact that this was unhealthy. Only now, years later, do I see how extreme my lifestyle was. I completely lost control before I could get a grip on the accelerating downward spiral. I truly thought that I was being "fit" and *getting* to the healthiest place I'd ever been, aka the perfect body. My desire for weight loss had originally stemmed from just wanting to feel like myself again. At first, I couldn't care less about abs. Then as the weight melted off, and I was so engrossed in that mindset, I felt that I *needed* abs. I wanted them and that perfect body so bad that I had no recollection of the fact that I was below the weight I wanted in the first place.

I had lost all sense of health and control was lost. Rigid, restrictive eating is the quickest method to that body, and that body equates to health, right? Wrong, and it soon became a way to cope with other things going on in my personal life. My obsession with losing more weight cost me friendships and deprived me of happiness. I may not have had a hold on those, but I sure could control my food.

I ignored my conscious mind and listened to my subconscious instead. It wasn't until I started my very own fitness Instagram account, which highlighted my weight loss, that I realized it didn't have to be this way. That it shouldn't be this rigid.

When I began to find more credible Instagram accounts that inspired me with messages of balance and true health, I had a major lightbulb moment. So many of those people had gone through what I was going through, and they eventually realized that being so strict and rigid all for a certain body is not at all healthy. It hinders you from living a life worth living by keeping you anxious and stressed over food, saying no to social events, spiraling further and further into negative mindsets and living the opposite of your absolute best life.

But you, my dear, you're reading this book. You WILL live your absolute best life ever! You're getting the tools and the know-how to start right now.

So here it is, let's start. Let's call out Edna's loads of lies and kick her out of the party.

There are two ways we're going to look at this. First, all of Edna's external lies she has floating around our everyday lives; and second, all of Edna's lies *we've deemed as true* internally, floating around our heads.

Exhibit A: Edna's external load of bull poop. Her messages are embedded in almost all the information we absorb on a daily basis. Juice cleanses and broader diets are just a couple of ways that our everyday lives have become so full of filth that it's difficult to see through it. This filth also shows up in the way we talk to strangers, loved ones, co-workers, and other human beings in general.

This is especially true with social media. Social media is a funny thing because it can be used for good; so many people use it to better the world. But it can also be so easy to become sucked into the comparison game, making social media quickly become a source of major negativity in our lives. We have the people on social media with the Edna-deemed "perfect body," captioning all of their photos with things like "I just ate pizza." Whether or not they really just ate pizza is beside the point. These messages floating around are what we absorb as the truth. For example, "She can eat pizza and have that body, I can't." Or the classic I loved to use, "She can eat pizza every day and look like that, I look at pizza and gain twenty pounds."

This isn't only for those who believe they're overweight. What about those who are thin and are told to "eat a cheeseburger," or "what do you eat, bird food?" Being teased because of your weight, whether over or under or just naturally thin, is not okay.

We are a product of our environment. Unfortunately, Edna is a bed-hog in her relationship with our environment and she likes to sleep sideways. Aka, all up in your business, all the time. Women are constantly being told we're not good enough, not pretty enough, and that other people are much more special than us. We look to others for external validation that we are good, smart, pretty, worthy, loved, included, and so much more. We fall into toxic relationships with the hope that this person will give us the sense of validation we are so desperate for. We meticulously manipulate food to create the most perfect body, becoming obsessed along the way because we think that *then* we will be pretty enough or good enough. In our careers, we work ourselves into the ground because it's the only time we feel validated or appreciated.

Listen. You could be the ripest peach on the farm and there's still going to be someone who doesn't like peaches. It all begins and ends within yourself. The only opinion that matters is your own. Ugh, I feel your annoyance through the pages again. "I've heard that a million times, but I don't believe that I am pretty enough, or smart enough, or *whatever* enough right now." Well, friend, hold onto your britches because it's about to get wild.

This brings me to Exhibit B: all of Edna's bull poop running the show in our minds. This is where Edna clouds our minds and makes us believe all of the horrible and invalid lies as truth *internally*. We see the external messages all over: the magazines, the TV commercials, in conversations with friends, co-workers, and family members. The messages then become so ingrained in our brains that we don't even recognize them as false or have the ability to form our own opinions about them because they have become our normal.

We are born with whole truths. We only eat when we're hungry. We find happiness in each and every day. We don't immediately find fault with ourselves. We don't look for comfort in putting others down, putting ourselves down, or justifying why we are better than others or vice versa. Over time, and by quite a young age, we begin to rewrite these truths into untruths that we believe to be true. Okay, that was confusing. Let me explain.

We are born with true beliefs (i.e., food is nourishment, not comfort; I am pretty, so is she). Then Edna shows up uninvited and we relearn these truths to form untruths (i.e., food is my best stress coping mechanism; she is better than me; I am not enough as I am to have an amazing loving relationship; I only get a raise at work if I work myself sick) and believe these as the truth. Make sense? Starting from a very young age and for the rest of our lives, we're in a constant internal battle just trying to make our dreams a reality. Making these dreams come true is quite a difficult task with all of these untruths floating around.

Alright, pause. I think you might be thinking I'm full of crap right now. You might be thinking, "I don't do this that often, I see through the lies. I form my own opinion." Oh, but do you? Let me share with you another story, one from my younger years. Let me show you just how intensely these messages cloud our minds, at every age, each and every day.

I grew up in a Disney-obsessed family. Like, obsessed in the strictest meaning of the word. I'm not going to lie, I'm sitting here writing this book with the sound of the Magic Kingdom train running outside my window. This is because I may or may not live right behind the Magic Kingdom as an adult. No, Disney World does not get boring, and yes, I do go every week. Okay, okay, sometimes more than once a week. But I digress. I was a Disney kid, that's for certain. The only television I watched, or even wanted to watch, was the Disney channel. My favorite books were about princesses and talking mice.

So where did my inclinations of being fat, ugly, less-than stem from? It surely wasn't television. At such a young age, where does this come from?

I was an adorable little kid if I do say so myself. My white blonde curly hair was done up and put together. Supermom always made sure I was dressed to the nines; looking adorable was my specialty.

I felt good about myself. I knew I was adorable, but there were a few instances in which it was subtly shown to me that I was chubby. This is where my beliefs of being less-than or ugly sneakily found their way into my innocent mind.

I was the youngest of all of the cousins in the family, so I was the easiest target to pick on. A few times, though, it was because I was chubby. A few of the cousins and I were playing Disney Charades (of course) in the living room. My sister pulled the card of the Fairy Godmother. She blew out her cheeks, mimicking someone more plump and began to walk as if she was a round shape.

"You're Diana!" my cousin yelled.

Supermom scolded him, "You don't say things like that. That is uncalled for."

Then I knew. I understood that I *was* chubby. I was easy to pick on.

But in so many ways, I was a lucky child. I had Supermom *and* Superdad. Every single day they reminded me of how special I was. How smart I was. How beautiful I was. My future was so bright. Lucky for me, those are the messages I focused on for the bulk of my childhood, despite the subtle "you're fat and ugly" from other sources.

A day was not over until Dad said, "Did I tell you I love you today?"

I'd shake my head no.

"I love you today," he'd say with that big smile of his.

To this day, out from under his roof he still says this when we're together.

So where else did I get these messages that chubby meant fat? And that fat meant ugly? That I was different? That I was "wrong?" My parents sure as H – E double hockey sticks did not teach me that, but these messages still got into my head, just in subtler ways. Sometimes the messages aren't as overt as telling a child she's fat and putting her on a diet, or telling them that they would be so much prettier if they would just not eat so much. Sometimes it's more indirect, like the way my cousin "suggested" I was fat, leading me to believe that when you're overweight, you're picked on and less than others. The point is, these messages come in all different ways.

That's the problem (okay, one of the problems) with the world we live in. We are so inundated with external messages regarding weight and body image. There are ten messages about body shaming for every one message about how to actually be a healthy human being. It's as if the media sees the next fad diet as important as President Trump's most recent tweet this morning.

Flooding our media and society with messages of *true* health, wellness, and fitness because it's *good for your* mind, body and soul is just not "front page worthy." Remember, extremes are easy—balance is hard. It's easy to get a rise out of people when the cover of a magazine says "Lose 20 pounds in 20 days." A headline of "Eat your veggies, and donuts sometimes too" is just too boring for us, or seemingly impossible and seen as a lie.

You see, my story begins on one side of the spectrum, travels to the other and ends in the middle. From being a chubby child eventually diagnosed with insulin resistance syndrome, to an eating disorder college, and finally, to creating a career as a health and wellness coach, spreading the oh-so-needed message of true health, nourishment, wellness, and body confidence. After experiencing the entire spectrum, I know how it feels to be at every single point. I understand the different perspectives within the difficult journeys people face.

As a child, small, subtle messages from people outside my immediate family brought me awareness of my weight. Nobody ever called me "fat." Nobody ever told me I was ugly, weird, needed to change, or less-than anyone else. I also didn't let it define me at that age, probably because I was too young to do so.

Then I grew into a pre-teenager. By that point, I'd let the message that I was the chubby one define me. I was no longer immune from the subtle innuendos that I was not as pretty as the other girls and that I needed to change.

During this time, Dad used to love to take me out to dinner. He loved to take the whole family out to dinner, but he especially loved to take my sister and I separately so that we got one-on-one time with him. Remember, he's Superdad!

We were at one of his favorite restaurants on Old Mission Peninsula in my hometown of Northern Michigan.

"What are you looking at for dinner, Di?" he asked.

As he asked me, I sat still, in full concentration counting out on my fingers how many things I'd eaten that day.

"Um, just the Caesar salad I think," I replied after noticing that I'd already eaten four things that day.

I was in middle school then, where kids getting teased because of their weight was normal. I'd heard plenty of the names the other kids had for some of the other girls in my class. I wondered, what names did they have for me? I wasn't about to find out or let it continue any longer. I was done being the fat one. I was done looking at the other girls and wishing I was more like them. So, I decided to change.

You know the first strategy that came into my mind to lose weight was? Eat less. Don't eat so much. Food makes you fat, so don't put as much in your body. My conclusion? Only eat the number of things I can fit on one hand. In other words, only eat five things in a day. "That will surely make me lose weight," I thought.

HOW ON EARTH DID MY INNOCENT TWELVE-YEAR-OLD SELF KNOW TO DO THAT? I have no idea. It terrifies me. Again, it was not my parents. It was not my sister. It was not the television I watched or the books that I read. Where on earth did I learn that extreme restriction was the answer? Hint, her name is Edna.

A few years before, around seven years old, I was a dancer. I took quite a few classes, so we were at the studio pretty frequently.

One Tuesday, I was in the dressing room at the studio getting ready for jazz class. I absolutely loved jazz class. Jumping and dancing around to fun music in adorable outfits, what more could a young girl want to do after school?

Getting ready for class, I overheard my friend Elizabeth start to cry, completely distraught and overwhelmed. She too was seven years old. I listened to see what was wrong, to see if I could possibly help her in any way. Then she mentioned the reason for her immense tears.

She'd just returned from ballet class. She was one of the best dancers in the class, beautiful actually, and she was auditioning to be on the pointe ballet competition team.

"You need to lose weight, Elizabeth. You're too heavy for pointe competition right now," the teacher had said.

EXCUSE ME, WHAT? Let that sink in for a second.

Let me paint the picture for you. Elizabeth was not chubby in any way. She was a great dancer, and already so passionate about it. What's more? SHE WAS SEVEN FREAKING YEARS OLD. Holy guacamole someone call the fire department this fires me up. She. Was. Seven. Years. Old.

After telling us what happened, she said, "But I've only been eating carrots every day, I don't understand why I'm still too big. I don't know what else to do."

Only eating carrots.

Seven years old.

No wonder eating disorders and disordered relationships with food and the body are so common. Not only common, but overlooked, almost ignored. No, not almost. Just ignored.

In fact, "Between 40 to 60 percent of children age 6 to 12 are worried about how much they weigh, and 70 percent would like to slim down . . . Approximately 80 percent of all 10-year-old girls have dieted at least once in their lives."[2] The majority of young girls under the age of twelve have received the message that they need to be smaller. They are unhappy with their weight and have tried to diet at least once. Picture a class of twenty fourth grade girls. Sixteen of them have attempted a diet. My heart aches. The messages of manipulating food and finding fault within ourselves have gone too far. We need messages of nutrition, healthy exercise, self-love, and self-care to overpower these devastating messages.

Before you know it, the topic of conversation at girls' nights will be how you need to lose fifteen pounds and how all you ate that day was an apple for lunch so you could fit this girls' night dinner into your calorie allotment. Why can't we just learn that some days we eat veggies and balanced meals and some days we have girls' nights when we drink wine and eat cheese?

Similar to when we go off to college, where drinking more calories than we eat becomes normal, almost expected. In order to be liked or considered "fun," you have to go out

---

2   http://www.nydailynews.com/news/national/diets-obsess-
     tweens-study-article-1.1106653

and get drunk every weekend, sometimes during the week too. To prevent the copious amounts of vodka and beer from creeping up our weight, the only solutions we perceive as available are to just eat less, purge, stop eating, over-exercise, or some combination of all four. Look around, that's what everyone else does. Why should you do any different?

I remember in middle school during recess one of the teachers would go walk the track every day. One day she invited us to go walk with her.

"Why do you walk the track every day Mrs. T?" a student asked during the third lap.

"I am working to get healthier and lose weight, and each lap around the track equals one M&M. I usually eat a few M&M's after lunch so I like to burn them off."

Food makes you fat.

Food needs to be burned.

We need to earn M&Ms.

M&Ms are something that make you fat.

If you eat M&Ms you have to make sure you burn them off.

Soon it becomes so normal that it gets into the ears of children, and the cycle repeats itself. These toxic messages become regular thought processes.

What about balance? Having veggies and M&M's too? Exercising because it makes you feel good, and it keeps you healthy?

I have a great friend and client named Julie who has grown well into her adult life thinking she was not meant to be happy, content, or loved. Going through years of abuse from family members, horrible relationships, and difficult life circumstances, food became the only thing that brought her comfort. After breaking up with an ex-boyfriend she went over to his home to pick up a few of her things after the break-up. He had a few people over for a party at the same time. As she drove out of his driveway he yelled, "Maybe if you lost some weight bitch you might be more attractive!"

Disgusting. Some people even get their sense of self-worth and validation by degrading other people.

Believe me now?

Oh, but by golly there is hope!

I am going to show you how to turn the recipe for catastrophe into a recipe for yippee. Okay, it's supposed to be "into a recipe for success" but that's the best I can do for my poetry skills. I tell you, I tried so hard but it's like rhyming with "orange."

While we can't control the external messages that Edna throws at our faces every day as if we're in an intense game of "pie in the face," we can control how we treat ourselves internally.

Let's get all up close and personal with you and your inner critic.

The words we use with ourselves are powerful. They are the most important words we will ever say. You know the saying, "You have fat, you are not fat. You also have fingernails, but you are not fingernails." Let me tell you, this phrase used to drive me up a wall and then back down it. BONKERS I TELL YOU. But now I understand.

How many times a day do you degrade yourself? Talk

yourself down? Neglect yourself? Negate a compliment? Would you talk to your three-year-old daughter that same way? Your best friend? Your mom? Probably not.

Start to become aware of how you talk to yourself. Notice when you say things like, "I'm so fat," "If I could just lose five more pounds," "I'm just not smart," or "I always attract heart-break relationships." You see, the mind is like your Aunt Patty who believes that unicorns exist in Australia— so darn gullible. What you give power to in your mind is what runs your thought patterns, your beliefs, your actions, and therefore your life. We are basically a bunch of sponges walking around absorbing everything in our environment (thanks Edna), creating beliefs from it (true or untrue), acting on those beliefs, and creating our lives as a result. The kicker is in the belief creation, rooted in our thoughts and words.

Begin to talk to yourself as if you're talking to your daughter. When you say things like, "I'm so fat, I feel like a whale today," would you say that to your precious daughter?

Also, how do you make these things true for yourself? Maybe later in the evening your stress relief comes from eating an entire bag of popcorn. The problem with this is how unkind we are to ourselves as we do it, and what we consistently tell ourselves becomes a self-fulfilling prophecy.

"Well, I've been trying for months to lose ten pounds and my weight hasn't budged, I might as well just accept I'm going to be uncomfortable forever."

"I've been eating so good all day, I deserve this pint of ice cream."

"I'm so burnt out, all I want to do is eat."

Or what about, "When I lose the last ten pounds, then I'll be perfect."

"Okay, well, I look okay after that ten pounds, but maybe five more will be better." Then five more melts off and you're still unhappy, feeling unloved, and like you still don't belong.

We believe these words as true and subconsciously make them true with our decisions. No, the simple act of saying these things doesn't magically pack on the pounds or leave us unfulfilled. It's the idea that we don't believe in ourselves. We convince ourselves we aren't capable of eating healthier, finding improved stress mechanisms, or truly becoming the ideal version of ourselves, so we don't even fully try.

Stick with me here, I don't mean to go all Negative Nancy on you, but there are just some hard truths that need to be brought to light. I know I've been pointing out quite a bit of negativity, and maybe it's caused you to realize how harmful your own thoughts or actions have been. But the good news is that by identifying and exposing them, we now have the opportunity to transform them! And transform them we will.

As you can see, my own formations of society's messages came implicitly. No one ever told me to my face that chubby is bad and the way to fix is by not eating. These messages and solutions naturally made their way to me through subtle messages and became truth in my mind. For others, this is not the case. Some people's parents put them on diets at a very young age. Others have been through incredible trauma and found a coping mechanism with controlling food.

We can't control what others do or say to us, but we can control our reaction to it. And you, my dear, are learning from my mistakes. You are becoming so full of truth, reframing your untrue beliefs into truths. You're not going to let Edna show up uninvited to your party. You're not going to let her and her posse in. You'll get your lie detector out and know exactly when she's a load of poop with a capital S.

Here's how.

1. Decide: If cauliflower can be pizza, you can be anything.

Pay attention. Get your notebook out, turn the music down. This is a big one. Do you hear me? Ready? Good.

Decide what you want. What do you want to accomplish? What is your goal in reading this book, or in life in general? Why do you want to be the healthiest version of yourself? Why do you want to be stronger? Why do you want more confidence? If you're saying, "I just want to lose twenty pounds," what do you think you'll have when those twenty pounds are gone that you don't have right now? Why do you want that? And why do you want *that*? Bring out your inner curious five-year-old and ask yourself why at least fifteen times.

Be honest with yourself. What do *you* want? Not what do your friends want, or your parents want for you, or what's cool these days. What do *you* want?

Your "why" should make you cry. If you're not a

blubbering mess with a box of tissues, keep asking why. Write it. Say it out loud. Believe it. Own it. Identify with it.

---

2. Learn: Nourish and flourish baby

You'll notice, Edna doesn't often bring her science books to the table. Believe it or not, nutrition actually has science built into it. Shocking, I know.

Create a foundation of understanding nourishment in every sense of the word. Keep reading here for more, but even outside of this book, make an effort to understand nourishment.

Carbohydrates are not actually little animals that crawl into your closet and sew your clothes tighter. Carbohydrates, fats, protein, and micronutrients all play a very important role in our bodies. From the amount of fat you hold, to your mood and your energy levels, they all play a lead role in the Opera that is your health, wellness, and life. When you take the time to see how to bring food onto your team (remember, you're the captain, you're in charge) and have it work *with* you, then you will see results and keep them. You'll also be able to keep Edna on the bench and stop letting her be a ball hog.

Write into your mental book of truths that nourishment is so much more than food. It is time with friends, phone calls with family members, time away from work, meaningful work, and anything that brings you joy, peace, or happiness. Believe it or not, taking time to act like a five-year-old at Disney World, shoot the breeze with your best friends at brunch, turn into Mr. Clean on the weekends, or do absolutely anything that brings joy and happiness into your life is also nourishment. Remember: mind, body, and soul. If you had a dollar for every time you read those words you could buy yourself sparkly new pair of shoes. Hey, I'm just trying to get you to remember it.

_____

_____

_____

_____

3. Become your biggest cheerleader.

I'm not saying become the person that no one ever likes to talk to because you turn everything into a conversation about you.

"Oh, there's a hair on your sandwich Shirley? I had a hair on my sandwich once. It was the most traumatic moment of my life. Let me tell you about it."

Don't be that person.

What I'm saying is that if you're constantly acting like the leader of the enemy army in your own internal battle, can you be surprised that your good side hasn't won yet?

Cut the crap.

Remember how important the way you talk to yourself is? Let's make some changes.

Now, every time you go into a room with a mirror do you look into it and lift your shirt and notice that those twenty bicycle crunches haven't brought a six pack yet? Stop doing that. Do you wake up and remember how unruly your hair is and decide you might as well not even try today? Do you see that your skin is acting up again, might as well hide in the closet all day? Have those five pounds you haven't lost become all you see when you look in the mirror?

STOP THAT.

Look in the mirror and say, "Oh, hello, beautiful. Let's have a fabulous day." Life is not all rainbows and unicorns all of the time. There are going to be bad days, plenty of them, but finding kind words for yourself will be your superpower in these moments. Remember that it's a bad day, not a bad year. For every negative, there are plenty of positives. Make the conscious choice to emphasize the positive.

Believe in yourself. You are the only one that can take your dreams and make them a reality.

Create a list of powerful affirmations.

"Seriously, Di? Affirmations? Have you lost your marbles?"

No, actually, I have not. I used to hear that and think, "Oh, it's the woo-woo nonsense again." Well, let me tell you, those woo-woo folks are onto something. At the beginning of my entrepreneurial venture, I heard that I needed to start repeating affirmations to myself. After I heard this from approximately 33.7 people, I decided I'd stop thinking I knew better. I listened and give it a shot.

Starting a business is a no easy task. If you put yourself out there as much as you should, you get rejected almost daily, especially in the beginning. Remember, I went through my fair share of self-empowerment and improvement, so I was pretty good at talking nicely to myself, but this was a whole new level. So affirmations it was. I began to write them all over the place, in my planner, on sticky notes, in my phone, on my bathroom mirror. One I wrote was, "I will create $6,000 this month," which is not an easy task when you're starting from scratch. Want to know what happened? Of course you do. I made $6,000 in one week.

"Why have I not been doing this since birth?" I thought.

Here's the dealio, though. When you create these affirmations, you can't just robotically write them down and hope that all of your wildest dreams just start dropping from the ceiling as you watch reality TV on your couch. Bummer, I know. The point is for them to be constantly running in the front of your mind instead of getting lost in the sea of all of Edna's bull poop you've been storing back there.

When you create these affirmations, pick some that are directly in line with your "why" and create a strong emotional connection to them. I make at least one for each area of life (refer back to the key areas of life in the introduction). You probably won't believe them at first because you've spent your whole life as the leader of the enemy army in your internal battle, so it's going to take some time to start believing the truth and unlearning the years of lies. It will probably feel awkward at first. Everything is uncomfortable, until it no longer is.

Here are some examples to get you going:

- I am happy, healthy, and confident.

- I am strong, beautiful, and a light to be around.

- I feel happy, healthy, and peaceful every day.

- I create my dream life.

- I am powerful and conquer any goal I set my mind to.

- I am a sexy son-of-a-gun.

- I am fly as hell.

Or whatever tickles your fancy.

_____

_____

_____

_____

4. Forgive and thank yourself.

Throw around the F word like you're the biggest rapper on the hip hop station of Sirius XM, and by the F word I mean forgiveness. You've spent years putting yourself down, finding fault, always feeling like you need to do more, be more, achieve more, you're never enough.

Maybe you've spent years using food as your best stress coping mechanism, or maybe finding fault in yourself has helped you feel like you're making others happy by putting them above you. Perhaps you feel like a loving person by always putting others before yourself, or, you've won the national comparison championship. Maybe you find fault in others to make yourself feel better. Whatever it may be, these are usually our minds' natural tendencies to make us feel better or attempt to bring us happiness. No wonder it's been so hard to override these thought patterns.

Thank that part of you that's trying to keep you happy, safe, and belonging. Forgive yourself for trying so hard while using the wrong mechanisms. Forgive yourself for thinking Edna was your best friend when in reality she's a lying, cheating, witch of the bunch.

You're pulling an emotional 180 here, step by step. You're up-leveling your thought patterns and processes. You're showering yourself with a newfound love and respect. Here you will find better replacements for your coping mechanisms and ways of making others and yourself feel happy, loved, and worthy.

5. Run the subtitles.

Let's say you want to watch a PG-13 movie but your eight-year-old refuses to move from the seat right next to you on the couch. Subtitles it is.

Your thoughts are your internal subtitles. Act as if your eight-year-old daughter is reading every subtitle that comes across that TV. Would you want your daughter to read those? Would you want her to think it's okay to talk to herself in that way? Would you want your daughter to think it's okay to talk about other people that way? I'll admit that I need to take a dose of my own medicine on this one sometimes. It can be tricky after years of PG-13 and R-rated self-talk.

Maybe if we could actually do this, young kids wouldn't go around asking our adult friends why they don't have any hair in the middle of their head. Embarrassing.

My point is, you've got to start thinking and speaking to yourself as if you are your own child, in the most loving way possible. Believe in yourself with every ounce of effort you can muster on the good days, the bad days, the days that poop hits the fan all day. You. Are. Powerful. You *will* create the health, wellness, body, mindset, confidence, the life of your dreams, and whatever the heck other things you desire that will help you contribute to living your best life for yourself and others. It's unrealistic to say that 100% of the time we can get rid of the negative self-talk, but *intentionally* making the effort is the important piece.

When negative thoughts *do* come up—because they will—it doesn't mean you are wrong or bad or not good enough. It takes effort and time to override these natural thought processes. As humans, our natural thought pattern tendencies are actually negative. "The brain reacts more strongly to stimuli it deems negative. There is a greater surge in electrical activity. Thus, our attitudes are more heavily influenced by downbeat news than good news[3]." Bummer right? So, for every positive thought you create, my dear, you are creating success.

Continue to become so in tune with your thoughts and actions that you begin to see when the negativity party is

3   Psychology Today.

coming, prevent it from happening, and continue on being your best, unstoppable self.

Run those subtitles until you know longer need them. Watch your life begin to be joyful, fun, and exciting.

6. Clear it up.

How many social media accounts or TV shows do you watch that bring you down? How much of your closet is full of clothes that make you feel like you're not good enough, not pretty enough, or fill in the blank enough? How many of your friends make you feel unsupported, pick on you, or find fault in you? This is a short tip, but a very important one. Get rid of anything that fuels the negativity. You don't need it anymore.

As you can see, Edna creates a lot of baggage that we don't need to carry. These action steps may be difficult, they may sound unlike anything you've ever done, but darling, you were made to thrive. Buckle up and get going. You've got this!

CHAPTER 2

Edna and Helga.
The dynamic duo.

"I'm sorry, what did you say? All I can hear is bullshit."

—Your response to Helga.

M Y DINNER GOAL at five years old? Be a part of the clean plate club. The more I ate, the more praise I got. My favorite breakfast? Tough choice, but it was a tie between breakfast pizza or when the school was selling Krispy Kreme donuts. Afternoon snack? Soft pretzel with cheese. Favorite lunch? When we'd pick up McDonald's and have it brought to school. Saturday routine? Dad took sis and I to the mall for a few hours to give Mom some free time, followed by K.B. Toys (does anyone remember that store?!) and either Chinese food or Taco Bell for lunch. Sesame chicken or taco supreme to be exact. My claim to fame? Being allowed into the local steak restaurant with a "no children under eight years old" policy when I was six years old because Dad told them I'd order a full rack of ribs and eat them all, and that's the truth.

This was my childhood. I grew up during a time with little awareness about food and nutrition, especially the effects of processed foods on our bodies and our health. During the late twentieth century and early 2000s, the U.S. was on a roll: cheapening our food supply, lengthening shelf life, creating what resembles an addiction to food, and a lacking in nutrition knowledge. "Chemical agriculture became widespread after World War II. Natural and organic farming methods were replaced with the use of chemical fertilizers and pesticides. The 1950's saw a boom in processed foods mainly due to the invention of the supermarket. Our grandparents and parents got to ride the wave of resilience passed down to them from previous generations. They could handle a certain amount of processed foods and environmental toxicity without seeing as much of an effect on health as we see today[4]."

During the late 1900s and early 2000s we didn't understand what adverse effects heavy processing would have on our bodies or our health. We ruined our natural insulin response and increased the likelihood of man-made diseases like diabetes and heart disease by making processed foods a regular staple in the American diet. More about this in a later chapter. Note, occasional bouts of processed food

---

4   Whole Food Nutrition, (wholefoodnutrition.net).

are okay; it is the regularity that rewrites the body's processes and begins the formation of disease.

Here's the dealio, though. My Mom and Dad (most likely yours too) did not have an understanding of this. Health and fitness weren't as important to our country as they are today, so these habits of fast food and processed snacks were considered normal. Supermom and Superdad had great intentions, but they were uninformed about nutrition and how to eat healthier.

At first glance, you may be saying, "Well, alright, just start to eat healthier once you know better." Ah, I wish it were that easy. We as humans are actually programmed to make things way more difficult than they should be, starting in early childhood. Cue the subconscious mind, the one that tells your inner critic what to say.

The subconscious mind is the backseat driver of your life.

"Don't go after that career you're not qualified enough. You can't get a better relationship than this. You don't deserve to find a happy healthy lifestyle, that's too much for you."—Your dumb-as-heck subconscious.

Your subconscious mind is also a big fan of Edna. She's got posters of Edna all over her room, never misses her new podcast, and praises everything she has to say. She takes in all of Edna's bull poop as dogma from a very young age. Therein lies the reason we take all of Edna's stories at face value and implement them in to our everyday lives without batting an eye. We are so *used to* being inundated with these stories that the subconscious makes us believe it as the truth.

But good news! As soon as we recognize these patterns and old beliefs, with some effort and hard work, we *can* change them.

Do you recall the days when you were about fifteen years old, learning to drive a car all on your own? And to get your learner's permit you had to drive with an adult in the front seat for a required number of hours?

There you are, driving Dad's sparkly first love on wheels and you're about to make a left turn when Dad screams, "SLOWER! THERE'S A CAR COMING OH MY GOD WHAT ARE YOU DOING TRYING TO GET US KILLED?" In reality, the car is a mile away and actually turning into the gas station posing absolutely no threat. Also known as, the back seat driver of the year. Well, that's exactly who your subconscious mind is. While we're at it, the subconscious deserves a name too. Helga? Sounds fitting. We shall call her Helga.

It's nine a.m. on the sidewalk of bustling New York City. The pace is high, the energy is high, and there's a sense of "we're about to get shit done today" in the air. Everyone is taking larger than normal strides because, you know, in New York you walk with a purpose, even if there is no purpose. The business men and women look fabulous in their freshly pressed suits and chic leather briefcases. Waiting at the stoplight, you hear the man in front of you in his late thirties, obviously on his way to a corporate office, say into his earbuds, "I don't know Sharon. I couldn't find my blankey last night. I just didn't sleep well. Talk to me after my nap." Then the woman next to him dressed in the fabulous designer suit says into her cell phone, "You know what Dave, the finger painting you wanted me to do yesterday was just too hard. Why do you expect so much from me?"

Weird, right? Very.

We are all like children walking around in adult bodies, trying to make decisions with our adult brains but ultimately following through with decisions from our child-like selves.

In the self-growth and personal development world, the subconscious mind (some call it the ego but here, we call it Helga) is talked about quite frequently and for good reason.

Helga causes us to make decisions based on limiting false beliefs about ourselves and the world we live in. She controls our emotions, beliefs, perception of reality, and decisions. Helga is created and instilled as truth during our infancy and into early childhood years. Through our experiences as children, we make decisions about ourselves, our reality, and the world we live in with Helga's input. And because Helga is a whiny five-year-old, she constantly needs validation from outside sources and acts based on fear of anything and everything. Helga has a funny way of keeping us nice and safe in our old comfort zone of, "I am never going to be the goal-getter, or the person who lights up a room when she walks in, radiating health, happiness, and vibrancy from the inside out." Helga likes to blame our circumstances on outside sources, living in victim-mode. She operates based on past beliefs and fear of the future and is not connected to the present moment. She is in constant fear of death. Seriously, she's dramatic.

The subconscious runs our life with ideas based on childhood stories and shows up in our adult years as Becky with the good hair looking to be validated by the scumbag men she dates. Or Alfonzo who loves to talk about all that's wrong in his life looking for validation from someone to tell him he's worthy of more. Or Shirley who works fifty-hour weeks and volunteers ten hours with four kids, never leaving a second of time for herself. She's learned that deserving money or appreciation comes from first proving it by working yourself into the ground.

Quite the drag, right? Helga and Edna get along quite well. This is the one and only time I think a reject table would be appropriate and there are only two seats: for Edna and Helga. Hopefully by the time it's their turn for the buffet there's no food left and definitely no party favors.

Oh, but the truest and best version of ourselves, often called your "higher self," knows what's up. This part of you holds the ultimate faith in you, in the universe, in your higher being, and operates with the truth of the world around you in the present moment. That truth is that you are capable of absolutely anything you desire in this world. You deserve a life confident as heck in your own skin, allowing yourself to feel self-love, appreciation, belonging, and worth every day. Confident in your own beauty to tell Sir-Flex-A-Lot that he's a poop-head and you're done dating him because he treats you like a second choice. Your higher self believes you hold all the power to make it so. This part of you lives in the present and finds validation from within. It believes you are loved, you belong, you make good decisions, you know what's best for you, and you have purpose.

This part of you sees Helga for what she is: a worry-wart who needs to shut the heck up. Your higher self is not stuck in your own head of lies and self-doubt; it believes in every single dream, goal, or desire you have inside of you. It also gets to work and makes things happen, but this part of you can only create this future *when we give it the power to do so.*

Your "story" or your life experiences that form Helga are what create your adult biology. Simply said, all the things that have happened in your life since infancy are the "stories" that have created the qualities of the physical and spiritual person you are today. From these experiences, we create beliefs about ourselves, the world, and reality. These beliefs aren't necessarily true, but we hold them as the truth in our subconscious minds.

This is why it is so darn hard to rid ourselves of bad habits and have the belief and faith in ourselves that we are capable of creating our dream body, health, mindset, and life. Humans naturally choose familiar discomfort over something new that could be life-changing because it takes work, it's different, and it doesn't feel comfortable. We like to stay in places we know, no matter how miserable we might be. For example, parting with your daily dessert at three p.m. that brings stress-relief, comfort, and relaxation is all sorts of difficult. SHOOT! But, hey. Not for you, friend. I've got your back. This is my specialty!

There are a few ways that Helga causes us to grow into adults with habits we hate but just can't seem to ditch. I am going to show you plenty of these in hopes to help you identify what might have been your foundation of limiting beliefs. That way, you can identify those little buggers and take the megaphone away from your backseat driver ASAP and start living your best life ever.

For some of us, at a very young age, our subconscious

rewrites stories about our beauty and our ability to love the skin we're in. It rewrites our understanding to nourish ourselves with real, high-quality foods because we truly want to, as well as our desire to exercise because it feels good. These new stories tell us we're not beautiful unless we have the perfect bodies, that food is something that makes us fat or covers emotional stress, that we can't create the confidence we want because it's not in our makeup, or that we can't become a thriving interior designer because there are too many good ones already.

Our parents likely instilled food habits from the beginning, like the ever-popular food-as-a-pacifier that begins as a toddler or even infancy. When you were two years old, maybe mom's go-to for making you stop crying when you were upset was a snack. Helga says, "food = no more tears or discomfort. Food = comfort and relief." So we form this belief that food is the best stress reliever or mechanism to numb whatever is currently bothering us. Thirty years later, the dramatic-as-ever Helga refuses to update her methods and stress-eating is as normal as breathing.

By this point, you're pretty familiar with my childhood story about food. My nutrition was not good, but it was normal to me to eat only what tasted good regardless of whether it was nutrient-dense and I had no understanding of the 80/20 rule. No wonder I wound up with insulin resistance syndrome at such a young age, eh? Being much bigger than other children, combined with my horrible diet that I found enjoyment and comfort in, and the fact that this was all I'd known for the bulk of my childhood, was what created a horrible relationship with food in my later life. By the age of twelve, with fear of going back to being the "big one" of the group, I developed the belief that if I ate less-than-nutritious-foods, I would end up back where I was as a child. More about how this sent me to the other side of the unhealthy eating spectrum during college in chapters seven and eight. For now, my childhood.

As I mentioned, the message that I was "fat" got inside my head as a child in various subtle ways. I had this darling act I used to do to get a laugh out of people, telling a joke so they didn't have a chance to make fun of me first. When I did it, I noticed it put a smile on others' faces. I'd put my hands to my cheeks and squeeze them while saying, "My mama said fat people can't smile, but I'll show her,"and I'd give my widest grin while squeezing my chubby cheeks. It was a guaranteed laugh. Everyone thought it was hilarious, and I did too. Looking back, the reality is that I was creating a laugh at my own expense, even if that wasn't anyone's true intention. Eight-year-old version of me thought I was just being the cute little stinker everyone loved me for. The adorable and chubby one of the family.

What I didn't recognize was that this was another example of the exposure I had to the fact that I was not like the other kids. I was not small. I did not have a tiny flat tummy. My cheeks were adorably more plump than other kids. My spine did not stick out like most girls. I was the cute chubby child. My identification of myself was that I was big and that's how everyone saw me.

I have another friend, Megan, whose parents put her on her first diet, the Atkins diet, at age nine. Her mother was a chronic dieter, always unhappy with her own weight and body image. As a result, she did not want her daughter to go through the same things and she projected her own unhealthy relationship with food onto her. So they both began the Atkins diet when my friend was just nine years old. Consequently, Megan's truth became that she is only pretty enough, good enough, or healthy if she was on a diet—that she could only have a desirable body if she was on a diet, always getting smaller. It was not possible for her to eat what she loved and as much as she wanted. She couldn't be in love with her body in her own skin and be truly confident without first going on a diet.

Parents are often coming from a place of love, only wanting the best for their child, as did Megan's. But as a product of diet culture, this approach only creates more trauma and unhealthy relationships with food and the body. Like Megan, some people are raised with the belief that food is the enemy, something that makes you fat. This creates a stress and anxiety from a young age that is brought into adulthood and seems normal.

And then my friend Julie. Julie is one strong, powerful, and incredible woman that I had the pleasure to coach through her emotional binge eating. Unlike me, Julie experienced trauma, abuse, and heartbreak the majority of her life.

We were always struggling from what I can remember. Mom always made us good, hearty dinners. They were very large portions, but it was all I knew so I thought it was normal. With our already larger than normal portions, overeating was easy and almost expected. It made me feel good, like a nightly comfort. I didn't notice I overate until about age nine or ten when I would hop on Dad's lap and he'd say, "Honey, geez, you're like a bag of bricks." Through years of abuse, bullying, and my own self-destructive thoughts and beliefs that grew as my body grew, I later understood I was numbing out and avoiding emotions with food. All my life I've turned to food for comfort, especially when I wasn't even hungry. It's like I'm on autopilot. And today, it's become such a natural response I hardly even know when I'm doing it.

After years of Julie's best coping mechanism being consuming large amounts of food, it became terrifying to let it go. Looking for a better coping mechanism and following through with overcoming emotional binge eating is arguably as difficult as breaking an addiction. It may take years to realize that you're using food as a coping mechanism because of how Helga has disguised it as the only answer. But if this is you, you're not a failure. You're not weak. You're human. It is possible to ditch this belief. It takes hard work, especially inner work, but it is so possible. Stay strong, and keep reading.

And that's where the pattern begins. From a young age, we are flooded with misinformation, quick fix fads, and messages that we are less than or not as good as other people if we don't have the "perfect body." We grow into our adult years believing them as truth. We struggle through our adult years desperately looking for the holy grail of, "I'm finally good enough as I am, in a body I am proud of and confident in, with the stamina to play with my four little angels every day after school, and the tenacity to turn my quilting hobby into a full blown side hustle that pays for our annual trip to somewhere beachy." But we have Helga on our left shoulder with red horns telling us we don't deserve that life, we're not made of that clothe, that's for other more qualified people.

Soon we can't even hear our higher-selves on the right shoulder with the glowing halo telling us we are powerful and deserving, that we were created to have that life, telling you to start believing in yourself and stop letting the lies and fear win.

It's not that those awesome humans who have identified their false beliefs, rewritten them, and begun to live their best lives never get brought down by their version of Helga anymore. I wish that were true. But the reality is, those of us who *do* identify Helga and her false beliefs gain a strong sense of what they are, what they sound like, what they feel like, and when they come up so that we can identify them as the lying bastards they are and continuously choose better beliefs instead. I'll show you just how to do this as well. Then, my dear, you will know exactly when you need to choose a better belief and get to keepin' on living your best life. Kapeesh? Goody.

After gaining my freshman "begin to eat like an average seven-year-old" weight, I mean freshman fifteen, my default mechanism to lose weight was to eat less, an idea I had formed as a young child. I defaulted to being restrictive, rigid, and strict. After the subtle messages I received, I formed these solutions as a young child. My subconscious witch with a capital B had zero faith in the fact that balanced, healthy lifestyles existed. My childhood taught my version of Helga that eating anything less-than-nutritious would cause me to be the chubby one, give me grief, and bring me right back to where I was as a young child.

Most of us grew up in diet culture. It was especially prevalent during the time of my childhood, where fat free, sugar, free, low carb, zero calorie became the end all be all for how to get healthier. For other children like Megan who went on Atkins at nine years old, they grew up in a household where their mom and dad were always on a diet. They were always trying the next best thing to lose the weight. Some might have been more extreme, where mom or dad constantly had disordered relationships with food too, obsessing about having the "perfect body"—always saying no to anything but salad because they ate bread yesterday, trying to lose the last ten pounds, or restricting because they have a party coming up and want to have dessert there. Maybe they told their children they're fat, they need to not eat so much. Are you picking up what I'm laying down? They end up passing these thought processes and beliefs onto their children.

There you have it. Your story creates your reality. Helga is a big hairy monster, especially when she teams up with Edna.

You're reading this book, though, so you must have the amazing goals of becoming the healthiest and best version of yourself. You're ready to break free, create your dream body, mindset, health, confidence, and ultimately your dream life. Hop to it, sister.

The perfect process to identify Helga's B.S., rewrite your story, and begin your dream life today:

1. Who am I?

Take an inventory of your childhood.

What is the story *you* grew up with and identify with today?

How did your parents/loved ones treat you as a young child?

What is the common denominator of your nutrition habits? Your exercise habits? The beliefs you have about yourself?

_____

_____

_____

_____

2. What is actually true?

What do you KNOW to be true, as opposed to the stories you've identified with since childhood?

Do you know that you are worthy and capable of having a healthy body?

Do you know that you are deserving of love regardless of what size your jeans are?

Do you know that you CAN have some french fries every now and then and be happy and healthy?

Because you are worthy, deserving, and you can.

_____

_____

_____

_____

3. Up-level the B.S.

When you envision the ideal version of yourself, what does that version of you embody?

Will you feel in charge of food?

Will you choose wholesome good-for-you foods because you *want* to and because they help you live better days?

Will you work out consistently, without being extreme, because you know it makes you feel better?

Will you be a light to the people around you?

Will you be the one people love to be around?

Will you be an entrepreneur?

Will you become a CEO at a large firm?

Will you no longer binge eat?

Will you eat foods you love without guilt?

By identifying the person your soul and your higher self knows you can be, and when you understand who you truly desire to be, you can then identify where in your daily life or habits Helga trips you up and begin to up-level with the tips and methods in this book. This way, you can finally put some duct tape over Helga's big mouth. Aggressive? Maybe. Necessary? Absotively posolutely.

---

4. Own it.

Get crystal clear in step number two—what is actually true.

Then own it, identify with it, and keep it with you at all times.

Write it down over and over.

Be the one with sticky notes everywhere and reminders every hour on your iPhone.

Picture yourself living as the ideal version of you. What does it feel like? What does it look like? Where are you? Who are you with?

_____

_____

_____

_____

5. Environment audit.

Your environment will always be stronger than your willpower. That means that when we

intentionally set up our home, office, relationship circle, etc. for healthy behaviors rather than destructive ones, we don't actually *need* willpower, which will increase our likelihood for success.

Surround yourself with people who encourage you to accomplish all of your goals as well. The last thing you need is negative Nancy making you second guess anything you're doing.

Oh, and for the record, people who are really good at listening to Helga have a hard time watching people shush of their version of Helga. It's hard to watch someone do what you deep down want to do but don't know how. You might get some haters, but don't worry. Their hate is not about you. They're trying to figure out how you got the confidence you now have, to go after what you truly want.

Do all of your friends make fun of the people looking to make a healthier lifestyle? It might be time for a few new friends.

Is your house full of your go-to binge foods? Clear the pantry.

Do you only follow social media accounts of people who make you feel inferior? Do some unfollowing. Follow people who lift you up.

Become friends with people who support of the life you want and are working toward their version as well.

Set up your environment as if you are the ideal version of you already. What does that look like?

_____

_____

_____

_____

6. Get shakin'.

Every single day act as if you already are the version of you who you are working to be.

How do you think?

What do you view as nourishing?

What is your routine?

How do you handle bad days?

Who are your friends?

What do you believe about yourself and the world around you?

Consistently CHOOSE to be this person. It's not an overnight change, I wish it were. Be intentional about trying your best to constantly choose to be that version of you in every single thought and decision.

There you have it. Childhood is a key role in the development of our adult selves with the formation of Helga. Often, it is a culprit for many of the bad habits we so desperately want to shed but find so difficult to do so.

It's not overnight, it's not a one and done kind of thing. But the more you practice, the easier it will be. It will be uncomfortable at first, but everything new is uncomfortable until it no longer is. Decide how bad you want it. Stand up more times than you fall down, and this time next year you'll be in a completely different place. Exciting, isn't it?

CHAPTER 3

There are plenty of fish in the sea, there's also a lot of pollution.

"I love you with all my butt. I would say heart, but my butt is bigger"

—A pretty funny anonymous person on the internet. Also me. I say this a lot.

D O YOU EVER feel like the stories in love songs are just fake? Does anybody really have that sort of love? I sure as heck have wondered this before, especially during college when every guy I talked to was either all house and no attic (Mom's way of saying handsome but dumb), or nice but boring, and awkward as heck. It's like that saying, "There are plenty of

fish in the sea. Yeah, well, there's a lot of pollution too."
Shootsky.

In this chapter, I'm going to lay it all down for you—the nitty gritty about romantic relationships, because they are a critical piece in the journey toward *true* health and wellness. I'm no relationship guru, but I'm sharing my story and the tidbits I have learned in an effort to connect with you and show you what you deserve in your life. Some relationships are incredibly supportive, and some are just plain old lousy. I was going to say "suck," but I feel like I shouldn't write that in a book, eh? Some are bad, got it?

I myself have a type: tall, dark, handsome, and male. But remember, if you're a fabulous guy looking for your prince charming, or a strong and independent woman looking for your lady, insert your preference in place of "guy, man, dip s**t," you get the picture.

Many of us tend to go about love in the wrong way. We think a new relationship will complete us, fill a void, and provide what's "missing" in our life. I get it, I thought that too. I thought about life in a sequence: you get the job, you marry the perfect man, you make beautiful babies, and you live a thriving life together with your white picket fence and labradoodle. And maybe you do all of those things, but let's first examine what's at the foundation of that idyllic love with 3.5 kids and perfect white picket fence. Even though I'm not a gambler, I'll bet you're wanting that relationship to fill your cup so that you're beaming happiness from ear to ear. Well, friend, that just might be the reason you're *not* beaming from ear to ear.

From a bird's eye point of view, being in the perfect relationship sounds like an ideal dream to have, but what about learning how to love *ourselves* first? Just like the need to teach true health, true fitness, and true wellness, we need to teach true love too. By loving ourselves, I mean feeling full and complete with yourself, 100 percent on our own. The addition of a life partner is just an incredible bonus. Kind of like going to Disney world right after you get off of a Disney cruise, you know?

You're here reading this book because you want to conquer your relationship with food and your body, or you want to finally feel like the healthiest version of yourself, or you're looking for the confidence to go after every single one of your dreams, regardless of others' opinions. That's magnificent. I am so proud of you. You will accomplish all of it. Romantic relationships are about getting *support* to do all of these wonderful things, receiving unconditional love in the process, and having a shoulder to lean on and believe in you in times of struggle. We spend a lot of our time with this other person, our partner. It's so easy to get lost in believing this other person knows what's best for you, or that their opinion matters more than your own. But the opinion of you that truly matters? Oh, that is your own, friend. This isn't new news, but you need to believe it, so I wrote it for you again.

Right now, I'm in the middle of planning a wedding with my soulmate. I prefer to refer to him as the prince charming to my fairytale, but I also wanted to mention he's my soulmate. "Here we go, another love story I don't believe in,"—your thought, just now. And I totally get that! But listen. Prince charming and I have had our fair share of bumps in the road to get to where we are today. It wasn't always like this, but *we made it this way*. We made it this way because we *are* soulmates. I knew from before we started dating that he was put on this earth for me—it's an unexplainable feeling. Somebody like that doesn't come around very often. We made our own fairytale despite the windy road it took to get there. Call me princess.

Aside from my husband-to-be, I've only dated one other person for an extensive period of time (we're talking more than six months and kindergarten doesn't count). But boy oh, boy, was that prior relationship meant to be in my life so that I could learn from it. His name was Nick—remember the one who came running back when I was in college? My relationship with him was hard as hell. I spent so much time trying to prove to myself that I could love him, even though I knew deep down we were not meant for each other. We looked good from the outside, so I was trying to believe we were good on the *inside* too. I exhausted myself trying to love someone who was not in love with the real me. The kicker? At that time in my life, I was struggling to believe in myself and what I deserve. My friendships were wavering because of my lack of confidence and struggle with body image, so I leaned on this toxic relationship with Nick which wasn't meant to last in the first place. I wanted to love myself, but deep down I hated myself. Not every relationship is meant to last. Some are meant to give you the lessons you need to become the person you're meant to be.

"Ethan said something pretty funny today," Nick said.

"What was that?" I asked.

"He said the best way to find a hot girlfriend is to date a girl that's kind of chubby when you first start dating. Then start working out with her until she gets really hot and then everybody is going to be so jealous. And I laughed because that's kind of like what I did with you," he replied.

"What?" I said, dumbfounded.

"Oh, come on, you were a little on the heavy side when we started dating again. I mean, look at the pictures from your sister's wedding," the dip s**t said.

"Yeah, I guess so," I said. At the time, because of my struggle to love my current body, I admittedly didn't think much of his cruel and naïve comments. I knew I'd gained weight during our freshman year of college. I didn't know how else to reply.

The first time Nick and I dated was senior year of high school. He was my first real relationship, my first kiss, and my first time trying to figure out how to not be awkward as heck in a relationship. Come Christmas time—about six months after we first started dating and on the day of my girlfriend's Christmas party—Nick broke up with me. I had seen it coming. He'd stopped responding to my texts in the lovey dovey way he used to and he stopped saying "I love you." I knew the end was coming. When he ended it, I cried for two whole weeks straight. I cried so hard I lost my voice. It felt like he'd taken a part of me.

But I eventually got over it. Then I went on to have the most fun I had ever had throughout my high school career, right at the end of my senior year. This is where my skinny jeans and crop top, raspberry Smirnoff and orange Fanta in hand type of confidence began and would continue through freshman year of college. I had broken out of my shell, or as my friend Brenna and I like to say, we jumped out of our shells.

As you know, during freshman year of college I was a

regular at the chicken tender bar of the dining hall, always down for a shot, dancing my tush off at any party I went to, and living the single life, if you know what I mean. Then came the summer after freshman year of college. After that year of freedom and becoming a little too much of a regular with fried foods, my confidence wavered again. As timing would have it, this is also when Nick came running back. He asked to get back together and I agreed, believing I was fulfilling the "relationship status" I should have had. In my low self-esteem and less-than-perfect body, he made me feel wanted. So began the most pivotal couple of years of my life.

Alright, pause. Let's have a little lesson here, shall we? If you break up with someone once, especially someone who treats you like anything less than gold, you probably aren't a good match, hence the break up. Take a long hard look before getting back together with an ex, okedoke? Okedoke. Back to the story.

Unsure of myself and not quite confident in my own skin, I was looking for someone to tell me I was pretty, even though I didn't feel pretty, valued, or special enough to be valued. With what I believed was my less-than-perfect body, Nick gave me attention and validation. I thought, "what if I can't attract anyone better than him, this poophead, if I never have a more desirable body? What if nobody else thinks I'm pretty enough for that sort of attention and validation in *this* body? What if no one else will want to be my boyfriend and not just a fun fling?"

Around the same time Nick came running back, another part of me had already determined I'd lose the weight I'd put on. Despite Nick wanting me back in my less-than-perfect body, I decided it was time I have my "best body."

Eventually, through my obsession with Pinterest, I'd do whatever it took to have the Edna-deemed "good" body. I started losing weight, even getting down to where I was before college, but I decided that still wasn't good enough. I needed abs, I needed to be tiny. After all, Nick was praising how tiny I had become.

A few months into being back together, sitting in his college apartment, Nick and I were talking about how I had finally taken some of my freshman fifteen pounds off. Remember his comment, "Get a girl who's chubby and make her lose weight?" Well, I'd lost the weight. I was darn good at restricting my caloric intake and getting more extreme by the day.

"I like it when I can see your hip bones," Nick said. They'd recently started to stick out more than they normally did, which made me feel accomplished.

"And you know when girls have those dimples on the small of their back? You should try and get those."

What he said felt good to my insecure self. I was finally becoming one of the skinny girls that guys love. For some, seeing your hip bones is natural. For me, it was a sign I'd gone too far.

After looking back, I can see how all I wanted was to feel loved and enough no matter what I looked like. Now? After learning to love myself and recognize Nick's comments for what they were? I'm disgusted. My heart aches for that version of me. I want to go back and show myself what was really going on. I want to show myself what's available to me in a relationship, what love really is. I want to show myself the freaking light.

I want to go back and say to Nick in that moment, "You

like it when you can see my hip bones? Do you know what that sort of statement does to a woman's mind? I am not a f**king dog. I am a woman. I deserve to be seen by my significant other as strong, beautiful in my own skin."

But that version of me didn't feel this way. She thought she was supposed to look a certain way to be enough for a "desirable" relationship. She didn't know how to truly love herself and stand up for herself. I thought, "Hmm, well, maybe I should try to make it so you can see more bones?" I had zero appreciation for my body, zero admiration for my own beauty. My worth and value were rooted in the idea that Nick needed to see more bones.

Extreme efforts to lose weight or achieve a certain look can result in neglecting relationships, work, school, or things that are supposed to bring us happiness. When we are only focused on a certain body type, it can make the path to true health much rockier. When the person who's supposed to love us unconditionally fuels that, the pathway out of it—towards true health—is difficult to find.

I don't believe Nick had any idea what power his hurtful words would have on me. He didn't understand the repercussions of what he was saying. He might not have been trying to make me hate myself or starve myself. But regardless of what he intended, his words broke me. Hearing his comments about my body turned my want for my pre-college body into a *need* for the "perfect" body. I needed abs. I needed to prove that I could look perfect. I'd do anything to be perfect.

No wonder it was so easy for me to fall for all the diet rules, diet culture, and extremely disordered eating patterns. Not only was my self-esteem low, but someone else was telling me that the extremes I was going to were *good*. With every pound lost, I felt proud for a solid sixty seconds, and then moved on to trying to make my weight lower. I thought that when I have the perfect body, I'd start to be myself again and be less strict.

I can tell you now that after years of inner work, throwing my untrue beliefs in the trash, and discovering *true* health, happiness, and confidence, I know what I (and you, sister) truly deserve. After fully loving and *nourishing* myself, and becoming 100 percent complete on my own, I found my dream man. I am 100 percent complete alone, but we're better together. And SHOOT. Let me tell you, all of those guys out there who tell you you're gorgeous and such a catch one minute then pretend you don't exist the next? They're from Jupiter and they only get stupider. They're also from mars and you should raise your standards bars. Okay sorry, this is not a poem. Stay on track, Di.

Envision yourself thirty years from now. Where do you want to be? What do you want to be doing? Most importantly, how do you want to be living? What I mean by living is, do you want to wake up on a Tuesday completely happy and excited to just live a normal day? To go to work, maybe the grocery store, cook dinner, and just be? Then to still be content, joyful, and in the absolute best place in life you could be on any given day? Feeling happy and healthy in your body, even proud of your body? Confident, beautiful, the best you have ever felt in your entire life? I don't mean to sound like Ms. Braggy Pants, but after years of hard work, this is my life now. It's not perfect, there are definitely bad days, but it's pretty darn great. And you can have a life like this too, friend. But how did I get to this fabulous place of being 100 percent complete on my own, only better with a smokin' hot man to do life with? Keep reading, my dear.

T, y forever man, my hubby-to-be. His name is Tyler, but let's call him T. Everyone

else gets a nickname in this book, so does babe. Shoot, that's another nickname. I'll stick with T. Recently, T and I were in Hawaii for a little vacation before he went into another intense year of Air Force training. Recently engaged, at dinner one night, we played one of those "100 questions to ask your partner before getting engaged" games. Well, the deed had already been done but we thought it could be fun anyway. Two questions and answers imprinted in my mind.

"Oh, this is a good one!" I said. "If we took away physical attraction, what would be left in our relationship?"

"A ton. We have so much besides that," he said, to which I smiled. I completely agreed.

"What if I gain a lot of weight?" the next question asked.

"I'd still love you the way I do now. I don't love you because you're beautiful, even though you are. I love you because of all of the little things that make you, you. You're smart, driven, passionate, even the way you have a short temper sometimes. It all makes you into the person I love. It wouldn't matter." Cue heart eyes and melty-gushy feelings.

He didn't say "you won't gain weight," "I'd help you lose it," or anything along those lines. Just, "I love *you.*"

That is love. Of course physical attraction is an important part of a healthy relationship, but if the other person makes you think you have to look like a swimsuit model in order to want you, hold it right there. Regardless of where you are on your health journey, intimacy should be fun. In a healthy relationship, when you slip your clothes off, he's not looking at what you perceive as your flaws, or your stretch marks, or your rolls. You know what he thinks? Oh, a booty! Boobies! Naked girl! If he makes you feel like you have to be a runway model before it's fun for him, consider how that is fueling an unhealthy relationship with food or your body.

For those of you already in a relationship, how do you know if it is helping or hurting your wellbeing? A relationship should give you the support and encouragement to truly be the best person you can be. To go for the goals that you find a tad crazy, but also exciting. To find happiness in the presence of another person on your worst days. Not to be your only validation. Not to remind you that you're good enough when you don't feel it for yourself. That's an inside job—one we'll discuss more in a moment. Validation, worth, enough-ness, beauty—these are all an inside job. Knowing and believing these things to be true in your own heart is a requirement for being able to completely love another person and to be the best version of you that you can be.

It took a lot of hard work for me to get to this place. So, back to the story. By the end of summer before my junior year of college, I was well-aware of my disordered eating habits and horrible relationship with my body. Instagram had become more popular, and I started to find balanced diet advocates who personally used to struggle with disordered eating habits as well. Up until this point, I just thought I was being "fit." I thought that's what it took to have a body like that. When I found these accounts, and people working to help others heal, I realized that what I was experiencing was not at all healthy. Rather, it didn't need to be like that anymore. Having a body you feel confident in and being able to live your life and eat what you want was a possibility, even a right. I'd never believed that for *myself* until then. I clung to my beliefs that I would not be able to have a body I loved without extremes. That is far from the truth, but oh how I wish it hadn't taken me so long to figure it out. I took it upon myself to work hard to turn it around. In doing so, I discovered a better version of myself, mind, body, and soul. I was able to clearly see that I did not need Nick in my life anymore, and I was better off without him. He didn't want me to have the life I wanted, and he was a major source of negativity.

When I finally broke up with Nick for good, I made a list of qualities I wanted in my future husband:

- Adventurous
- God-loving
- Loyal
- Compassionate
- Hard-working

I remember reading them out loud to my Mom and she said, "You know, you may have to compromise on some of those." "No I don't," I thought. I deserve to have someone with every single one of these qualities, and I trusted that God had a man with all of them for me. Now I'm with Tyler and he has all of those qualities. I didn't have to sacrifice a single thing. I just had to be strong in my beliefs and value of myself to go after everything I deserved.

Tyler had been a friend since I was seven years old. I'd always admired his adventurous spirit and determination to be the best in everything he did. After a year of not seeing each other during college breaks, just days before I broke up with Nick, I ran into T at the mall while home on break.

"I'm so happy to see you! What are you up to these days?" I asked.

"So happy to see you too! It's been fun being home, but I'm excited to get back to the Academy. I'm going to Germany in the spring with a group of other cadets to study and do some work with the Air Force. This semester my roommate and I are travelling over the country to do some business competitions with an agriculture company we started. And in our free time we're trying to visit all of the big ski resorts in Colorado! We're definitely trying to take advantage of everything we have available to us, it's been so fun. I feel so lucky," he said.

My heart immediately lit up. He was exuding every single quality I desired. He was going after life full speed ahead. He was taking advantage of every opportunity that came his way. He wasn't afraid to go after what he wanted. He was creating opportunity whenever he could. Then I knew— there are other people out there besides myself with the same zest and excitement for a truly amazing and adventure-filled life. I knew there had to be someone out there like that for me. Turns out, God wanted that person to be Tyler.

At that time, I was still doing hard inner work, learning more about myself and who I really want to be and making major improvements in every aspect. I went down the road to bettering myself for the entire year to follow. Tyler and I continued to talk after we saw each other at the mall that day, but I knew I wasn't quite complete on my own yet. I still had work to do.

During that time, I learned that love is an inside job.

I spent my spare time reading wellness articles, doing self-love practices, recovering from disordered eating, and repairing my relationship with my body. I desperately wanted to just be genuinely happy again. I wanted that carefree spirit of my younger self back. But friend, I was never strong enough to ask for help. How I wish I would have been, because my road would have been much shorter. I was trying too hard to appear strong and not admit to others that I needed help. I decided doing it alone was my only option (wrong). We'll talk more about this in the next chapter.

Regardless, I flooded my mind with self-love practices, affirmations, listened to endless podcasts on positive body image, true nutrition and wellness, how food works *for* you, how to align with and *be* the best version of yourself, and how to heal a broken relationship with yourself. I did so much work on myself that the new, positive messages filled my mind more than my negative triggers, but my path to healing was still incomplete. It wasn't everything I needed. It took me years longer to recover than it needed to. Always seek guidance, just like you're doing by reading this book. If you find yourself struggling like I did, don't be ashamed to ask for even more help, whether it's from a coach, a therapist, or a family member.

One way I did ask for help was through God. I asked Him to guide me. He guided me toward all of the self-love, and *true* wellness information I needed to heal. Although now I know I needed support from my loved ones, He will always be the first one I lean on when times are hard. Spirituality can be just as much of a helper as the next best self-help book and I am grateful for the courage He gives me to listen to Him. As always, substitute here for whoever you believe to be your higher power.

What I wish I'd learned at an earlier age is that you truly have to be 100 percent complete on your own before you can give yourself to someone else. So often people look for validation and self-love by hearing it through someone else's words, but we have to be able and willing to say it to ourselves first and believe it.

A partner should never make you compare yourself to other people. It's not that neither of you will ever have bad days or feelings of self-doubt, sadness, and so on. It's that you both support each other's goals and dreams, are confident enough in yourself to know when you or the other person is wrong and to admit to it, and love the other person wholly, not in pieces. During our younger years, it's so easy to ignore red flags and think we can change other people. You think they'll change, and you compromise your own desires in order to keep the relationships alive. What's missing is your relationship with yourself, the love and completeness you must feel with your own body and soul first.

Here are some red flags to look out for, whether you're already in a relationship or looking for one. Are you or your partner jealous? Are you or your partner constantly comparing yourself/themselves to other people? Never feeling good enough? Always afraid that the relationship might not last? Feeling like you have to always look or act a certain way? Be radically honest. These might seem obvious, but have you ever been truly honest with yourself about the answers to these questions?

When you can enter a relationship with the belief that

you are deserving of an incredible love, you know and are confident in your worth, then you have the ability to identify the things not meant for you and stand up for yourself when you need to.

At first glance, it may seem too good to be true with T. But I told you, things weren't always perfect. We went through a rough patch during our "kind of dating, but no label yet" time period. During that time, I thought our relationship might end for good. We (especially T) weren't the best version of ourselves. I wasn't as far along on my journey to self-love as God needed me to be, and He had a lesson to teach T along the way too.

It was Christmas break during our senior year of college. Tyler and I had been talking daily. We discussed the future, our goals, and found comfort in each other. We weren't officially together, but I thought we would be soon. I thought we'd go back to school after Christmas break as a couple. That day, still on break, I was sitting in the parking lot of the tanning booth around Christmas time of senior year (yes, I used to tan, emphasis on the *used to*), when my best friend called again for the second time. Somehow, my gut knew why, so I answered.

"Did you hear what Tyler did on New Year's Eve?" she asked.

"What do you mean?" I asked, scared of the answer.

She told me about the other girls, that I wasn't the only one. I was heartbroken, again.

But this time *I* was different. I had done the work to know and believe in my value as a person. I understood my worth—I believed in what I deserved and I wouldn't stand for anything less. What I know now is that God was testing me. He'd shown me down a difficult path to self-love and self-respect, and now He was making sure I understood.

After returning to school, fed up with Tyler's games, I stood up for myself.

"You're actually an asshole now, Tyler. You're done treating me like I'm worthless, I know I'm not. Your ego has turned you into a person I never want to speak to. The person you've become makes me sad," I said.

Defensive and full of excuses he responded, "Well, we weren't dating. I wasn't doing anything wrong. How am I supposed to know you weren't talking to a bunch of other guys? It's not all my fault."

Today, it saddens me to remember this time because I know the person he is deep down. He's the person I am now going to marry, not the one who used me that year. But if I had never stood up for myself and told him I deserved more, I would not be marrying him. In standing up for myself, I showed him that I demand respect. I showed him my worth, my value, and the strong and independent woman I am. If I'd never done that, he wouldn't have snapped back into the person God created him to be. He would've walked all over me and moved onto someone else. God put this in our story so I can prove to myself that I am worthy and deserving of an incredibly loyal relationship, and to straighten T back out onto the path toward the life God created for him.

Six months after I ended it with T during our rough patch, and after no talking whatsoever, God pulled us back together. It was clear that my words had affected him. He'd done some inner work of his own. We were both at the same gym at six a.m. one morning right after graduation from college. I had been studying for my CPA exams all summer, and Tyler had just returned from the Air Force Academy, so he was used to waking up early. We were the only two there—I believe it was fate. We spoke to each other and I could tell that T was back to his true self, the one I admired and adored. In the weeks that followed, we had honest conversations about what we both wanted. We've been together ever since.

Today, T believes in my dreams just as much as I do, sometimes even more. He's back to the person I knew growing up, and even better as we grow older. He makes me feel beautiful despite my cellulite (which is a natural thing to have), or when acne shows up, or when my body changes. He teaches me how to work endlessly toward every single one of my goals. He paints the vision of our future life and accomplishments with me. He's a role model for so many people. I could go on for hours about his tremendous support as a partner.

I know I never would've been able to love T in the way I do now, or even close, if I never went through my journey to loving myself.

We have to love people for who they are. If we want to be loved for the person we are, and the person we are growing into, we must give that as well. Do you love your partner for who they really are? Do they love you for you? Is there a part of you that is hoping they will change? Is there a part of you that hopes this is just a phase? Are you in love with the idea of that person, or actually that person? True and authentic reciprocated love is unconditional. It does not hope for change. This is probably not the first time you're hearing these things. But this time, I'm asking you to be genuine in your self-examination on this. If your answers are cause to be weary, then friend, your self-love journey is about to get deeper.

Most importantly, though, do you believe in yourself? Those passions that are so strong in your heart, do you trust you can make them your purpose? The dreams that have now become goals, do you believe you can achieve those? Do you know what you want in life? The kind of life you want, the marriage (or not) you want, the daily routines and things that bring you incredible happiness every single day . . . do you know all of these things for *yourself*? If the answer is no, how can we truly create our own best life if we don't know what we want? How can we love ourselves enough to create a body we're proud of if we're in a constant space of self-hatred and looking for someone else to love us when we can't love ourselves? If you're insecure with yourself, how can you create a healthy, loving, and thriving relationship with someone else? You simply can't give love to another person when you don't have enough for yourself. It's not about being selfish. It's about having self-respect and staying true to what you want in life. First things first, the answer to these questions must be "yes." Then, with this confidence and understanding, we can enter a relationship that is life-giving, instead of void-filling.

That's not to say that if you're currently in a relationship and not yet at your best in terms of loving yourself that you can't continue a thriving relationship with that person. Could you have open communication with that person and let them in on your journey to self-love and acceptance so you can bring yourself fully to the relationship? If that person fully supports you in whatever you want, how can you show up even stronger for them in doing the hard work to be your best self, 100 percent on your own?

When I was with Nick, I had goals and aspirations to move to a big city, work for a large accounting firm, and see how far I could go, but Nick didn't want that for me. He wanted me to be a stay-at-home mom, live in a small town, and have a mediocre life, never knowing how far I could take myself in my career. That's great for people who want that, but for me, his vision just wasn't aligned with my true and authentic self. And my gut new it. My intuition kept trying to tell me we weren't meant to be together. Nick was always fueling my sick relationship with food and my body, and I deserved to work toward my dream health, career, and life. Eventually I got the picture and said goodbye. It wasn't easy. It was a massive, terrifying leap. It meant finally acknowledging my strength and belief in myself on my own. It was a scary thing to face. Could I handle being alone? My heart told me I could, and God told me I needed to leave. He told me I was meant for a different life and my pathway to greater healing started with leaving Nick. Then I would be able to focus on myself, healing myself, and learning to love myself 100 percent on my own before allowing somebody else in.

Now, T supports me in everything I want to do, like when I quit my high-paying, cushy, secure corporate job to start a health and wellness business.

"So I've been thinking a lot lately, and I think I want to quit. I want to be a health coach. I want to help people discover true health and wellness and create their best life," I said, the nerves bringing me to tears.

"Wow, that's great. When can you do that? You would be so great at that," he said. That's when my tears started pouring. He was being supportive in the way I'd always needed. In that moment, I realized that God made him for me, and me for him.

"Seriously? I can't even tell you how grateful I am to hear you say that," I replied, a huge blubbering, sappy mess. His support was and continues to be unwavering. He could've questioned me, focused on money, or feared for our future. But he didn't. He believes in me and every single dream I dream up, and I do the same for him.

"I'm living my dreams every single day, you deserve to be doing the same thing," he said.

Unending support in every single area of life (health, money, career, relationships, spirituality) is what you deserve, friend. I know this sounds so foreign, almost impossible when you're struggling to accept yourself in your own skin—struggling to feel confident like you actually do deserve the world, or struggling to let go of your negative relationships with food and your body.

When struggling with disordered eating or abnormally preoccupied with weight, life can be lonely and isolating. Intimate relationships, whether it be a boyfriend, girlfriend, husband, or wife, struggle along with us in our bodily struggle. It's natural to want to isolate yourself in order to feel in control of everything happening such as the the food you eat, the exercise you do, and the environment you're in. Often times, our intimate relationships are not only hurt, but they fuel the fire.

Like with my experience with Nick. I pushed my
friends away, and I spent more time in toxicity. It felt safer
there, and I didn't realize I was contributing to it. Getting
yourself out of this situation is difficult. For months I
knew it was wrong, but I couldn't find the courage to get
out of it. I couldn't talk to my friends about it. I was lost.
If you find yourself in a phase like this, lean on faith and
love to know that your heart will guide you to what's meant
to be in your life. Trust your intuition. Have the courage
to get out of the toxicity. Your heart will show you the
bravery to begin living the life you were created to live.
Don't worry, we'll get real specific here so that you can do
this now.

I have a friend and client, Ashley, who is one of the
most beautiful people I have ever met, inside and out.
She came to me for healthy weight loss. Meaning, she
wanted to truly understand what methods are healthy,
what makes a food more nutritious than another, how
exercise fits into the mix, and she wanted to do it all
without having to say no to her favorite things like happy
hours and pancakes. She wanted to know how to create her
dream body. So that's what we did. Not by restriction and
deprivation, but through balance and *nourishment.* And
you know what? She re-discovered a sense of self-worth
and confidence she has ALWAYS had. Toward the end of
the program, we went through an exercise to tap into her
intuition and personal power. She'd recognized she'd been
lying to herself about her "perfect" relationship with her
boyfriend. Deep down she'd known it wasn't right. They
weren't meant for each other. On the outside, everything
looked great. She'd spent years lying to herself about what

she wanted in a partner, and she finally saw through her own lies and found the courage to go after what she really wanted.

When she re-entered the dating world, we discovered that strengthening her confidence muscle was a must. She's gorgeous, smart, has an incredible job, and her life was headed in a wonderful direction. But upon entering the dating world, she discovered she didn't believe this enough for herself and she fell victim to comparing herself to other women. She didn't have the guts to show people her raw and authentic heart, unable to give herself freely.

Through inner work—the same steps I am going to show you—and putting a system in place for her to consistently remind herself of her value, her worth, and everything she deserves in life, little by little, Ashley's confidence muscle is growing.

Another friend and past client of mine, Julie, struggled severely with binge eating. She'd experienced a lifetime of abuse, some even life-threatening, especially in romantic relationships. Her way of coping with her trauma was by finding comfort in food. We also went through these exercises to help her understand the self-destructive habits and build better ones in place of them.

Our stories are always different, but the unhealthy result is often the same. We fall into the trap of creating horrible relationships with food and our bodies, and distancing ourselves from what we truly deserve.

We subconsciously create what we don't want. With that in mind, take a step back and examine your own thoughts and actions. Who are you attracting? The subconscious mind, Helga as we know her, is always conspiring to make your thoughts true. Do you consistently say things like, "I suck at relationships," "I always attract the worst guys," "I'm just not good at dating"? Well, friend, you might be making that happen for yourself. If you *were* a good dater, how would you act? If you *were* good at relationships, what would you say, think, do? If you attracted *great* guys, who would you attract? Where our focus goes, energy flows. Set your focus on what you want, your confidence in yourself, and your own worth, and watch Mr. Right come walking into your life when he is meant to.

When you've established this unwavering self-love and confidence, you can truly love another. You can love someone so much that your happiness is directly connected to theirs. Your goals and dreams might seem so set in stone, but then you'll meet this person and your goals and dreams will amplify. They become even better and even more exciting.

Here are the steps you've been waiting for. This is how to set out on the path toward self-discovery and love and being 100 percent complete on your own. The steps to listen to your intuition, discover if your relationship is healthy, and find the relationship to help you create your dream health, confidence, and life.

Always begin with understanding what you need to do to start loving yourself, regardless of how you feel in your own body. Identify how your relationship with food or your body is unhealthy. Take action to tackle these first and foremost. Hiring a coach is a great first step. Some may need therapy, some may decide to get a gym membership and a positive body image book, and some may just need the support to begin taking action in a healthier direction. Whatever your story is, get to work!

_____

_____

_____

_____

1. Trust your gut, it always knows.

Our bodies are powerful. Our gut intuition tells us what's right or what's wrong. Deep down, if something feels off, it is.

Write down a time when your gut told you something was off, you followed it, and it was right.

_____

_____

_____

_____

If you're in a relationship, write down what your gut says about it. Write from your heart. Don't edit, don't overthink or second guess, just freely write. If you're not in a relationship, go to the next question.

_____

_____

_____

_____

Whether you're in a relationship or not, write down five qualities that you desire in a future partner. Look at your current relationship, are they there? Are you hoping they will change? If you're not in a relationship, when dating, seek these qualities out first and foremost.

2. What are your triggers?

If you haven't already, I encourage you to seek outside help, such as a coach or therapist, to help you go through these.

Identify your triggers. What are the circumstances that cause you to binge eat, restrict, or over-exercise? We'll cover these more in detail in chapter seven.

_____

_____

_____

_____

On the same token, what are your triggers in a relationship or while dating that cause you to feel inadequate, to compare yourself to others, or to feel jealous? What are the specific circumstances that bring these about?

_____

_____

_____

_____

Begin to notice when the urge to do these unhealthy habits arise, and what caused that urge. You will become aware of patterns and begin to see them coming. In doing so, begin to form new habits when these triggers arise so that you have a new plan in place for a better outcome. You can do so with the following step.

3. What would your ideal self do?

If you were already the ideal version of yourself—the person you are striving to be—what would he or she believe about your current relationship or the relationship you're looking for? What does the ideal version of you believe to be true about yourself, your worth, and what you deserve? How does this version of you act?

_____

_____

_____

_____

4. What do you truly want?

What do you want in your life? How do _you_ want to live? Not what your parents want for you, what are your friends doing, what's "cool" these days, but what do _you_ want?

Paint the picture, get nice and detailed, lay it all out. How do you want your life to look? How do you want to feel on an average day? What do you want to accomplish?

_____

_____

_____

_____

5. Is your partner helping you?

Does the person you're with (or if you're not with anyone, always keep these in mind) support your desires? Do they make you feel like you have to improve? Like you have to try and be like someone else? Like you're not good enough? Or do they make you feel extraordinary. Like you're a catch, and that they're lucky to have you? Listen. To. Your. Gut.

_____

_____

_____

_____

You deserve a love and partnership that makes even an incredible life look sweeter. A relationship where tough times are made even a little bit lighter, and where true support and unwavering love is a necessity. It exists, you deserve it, no exceptions.

CHAPTER 4

"In the age of the most connection outlets, we are the most disconnected."

"True Friends are like diamonds—bright, beautiful, valuable, and always in style."

—Nicole Richie

YOU'RE GOING TO live a fabulous life. What's even better than experiencing happiness in your own life, day in and day out? Having a lady gang to share it all with, or a man squad, or a wolf pack—whatever rocks your socks. Friendship. Your tribe. The people who build you up. One of the basic human psychological needs is intimate relationships and friendships, stemming from our physiological need of safety and security[5]. I'll take it one step further—a sense of belonging and love is a basic human right. We all deserve meaningful relationships that bring us a sense of love and connection with other people.

Can we all agree that an accomplishment, birthday, celebration of your first half marathon, or a bash to celebrate the fact you finally made cupcakes without burning them are all a heck of a lot more fun with other people who are just as excited for you? Especially if the cupcakes are chocolate with peanut butter frosting.

No matter what your dreams are, you need people around you. Say you're going to become the absolute best news anchor out there. Or maybe you're the next All-American basketball player. The next cake boss? The very best mother on the face of the planet? Whatever your big juicy life goals are, you're going to accomplish them. If you're going to make the most out of this life, you darn well deserve to have a tribe to do it with. A tribe that supports you in being the best you that you can be and brings the wine when there's a new season of the *Bachelor* starting, am I right?

Chances are, your lady gang, man squad, or wolf pack is going to change as you grow older, discover a deeper sense of who you truly are, and realize what you want to be in life. That's just how it's supposed to work. There's a theory that you are the five people you spend the

---

5   McLeod, Saul"Maslow's Hierarchy of Needs," Psychology Today, (https://www.simplypsychology.org/maslow.htm).

most time with. Meaning, you have the same mindset, values, motivations, and enjoyments as the five people you spend the majority of your time with. Naturally, as we grow and evolve and decide what life path we want to take, the people around us will change as well. We already know that some relationships are meant to last a lifetime, and some are meant to teach you a lesson (remember Nick? Of course, how could you forget). Powerful, right?

Sometimes the people we think are our friends tear us down instead of build us up. Betrayal, jealousy. Friendships, as important as they are, can also be challenging, especially for women.

Think about it, if a guy gets mad at his guy friend, usually it goes something like this:

"Hey, man, sorry about that. I was hangry and I took it out on you," guy number one says.

"Oh, yeah, I forgot about that. It's fine. Want to go to Buffalo Wild Wings?" guy number two responds. And then it's done. End of story. Finité. Is that a word? It sounds Italian for "finished" so I'm going to run with it. You wonder why my editor always has comments.

Girls on the other hand—six years later we still can't admit who was in the wrong for the fight we don't even remember the details of.

Why? Why does it have to be like that? Girls can be so mean, competitive, and jealous, especially when we're younger. Where does this all stem from? People loving the movie "Mean Girls" way too much and taking it too far? Nah. It stems from wanting to be loved. Wanting to feel included and cherished. You might be asking, "well don't men want and need this too?" Yes, but differently. In Emerson Eggerich's bestselling book, *Love and Respect,* he writes that "74% [of men] said that if they were forced to choose, they would prefer feeling alone and unloved rather than feeling disrespected and inadequate[6].") A man would rather know his friend still respects him than feel appreciated and loved, which makes this little Buffalo Wild Wings debacle make sense.

As women get older, our fear of not being included or loved grows, and often our only response is to prove why we are better than another. We might make fun of others. We might exclude people. We might pick fights to prove one is better than another. In order to be loved, we might go with the crowd. We might make decisions based off of what's cool, what will get us liked or noticed, hoping to feel a sense of belonging. Pretty twisted, right?

Oh, friends, what a blessing it is to have true friendship. What is *true* friendship? It's someone who will listen when you need to vent about how much of an idiot your boyfriend was last weekend. Someone you can call up when you're looking for a night so full of laughter you might pee your pants. This chapter is about finding and keeping them—your tribe. It's about finding the people who love you through your difficult moments and stick with you through it all.

---

6   Springer, Shauna H. "Women Need Love and Men Need Respect? A best-seller built on a faulty premise," Psychology Today, (https://www.psychologytoday.com/us/blog/the-joint-adventures-well-educated-couples/201210/women-need-love-and-men-need-respect).

It's about cherishing these friendships like they're a brand-new, six pound five ounce beautiful baby. It's also about uncovering how we naturally sabotage these friendships. How some friendships are meant to last until you're old and wrinkly in a nursing home together, while others are meant to be short lived, thankfully, and teach you a lesson.

You, friend, deserve to find happiness and love in every single day. On the days when it's difficult to find that happiness and love, you deserve to have your people bring them to you. It's challenging to go down the windy road to self-love—finding a strong appreciation for your body and learning to treat it as best you can—especially if you're coming from a place of self-hatred. Throw a lack of confidence or self-appreciation in the mix and you've got the best darn batter for some jealousy flavored vicious pie.

Bear with me. This is a tough subject. It's not rainbows and unicorns, which is why friendship gets its own chapter in this book. It is THAT important. I mean, didn't *Sex and the City* make that pretty obvious?

As we grow older, we tend to pick away at our flaws, finding "problem areas" and looking for reasons to diminish our confidence. In doing so, we often sabotage our relationships, especially friendships. I know I did. During college when I was struggling to find a version of my body I could love, I wanted to appear strong and in control. I didn't want others to know I was struggling. I kept my problems my own and never talked about them with anyone, even those I trusted. I isolated myself.

When going through disordered eating, or going too far with weight loss, isolation is a natural defense. "Isolation and eating disorders go together for many reasons. Often people find themselves avoiding situations where food will be involved because they are either afraid of overeating or they don't want deal with the questions or the looks if they are restricting. People also find that they begin pushing away friends, family, and partners in order to spend more time with their ED behaviors[7]."

My isolation began during college when I was a few months into my second relationship with Nick. I isolated myself from my friends when I was with him, retreating deeper into disordered eating. I felt like a bad girlfriend if I didn't spend most weekends with him, as if I had to be with him all the time. I didn't allow myself to be honest about what I really wanted in a relationship. From the outside, he appeared to treat me well and people told me I was lucky. I wasn't confident in my instinct that we weren't meant for each other or that I deserved better. I didn't believe that I could find someone who was truly made for me—who loved me for me, not my hip bones. I didn't think I'd find someone I could love in the same way I loved seeing the waitress coming with my food. Just kidding. But do you see? I lacked confidence in myself.

Little by little I was spending more time with Nick and less time with my friends. I was lost, but I couldn't see that. All I could focus on was my need to be skinnier or see my abs. I wanted control over my food, but I was losing my friendships, going deeper into a relationship that wasn't healthy for me. Losing closeness with my friends made

---

7   Binge Eating Therapy. (bingeeatingtherapy.com).

me feel out of control, so I continued to find comfort by controlling my food.

During my isolation, I felt the shift in my friendships. They were no longer as tight as they once were. My friends didn't feel love from me like they once did, and I didn't feel it from them. As my friendships crumbled around me, I felt like I was dangling from a fraying rope. I was further than ever from the tight friendships I once knew.

One night during this period of isolation, my three roommates and I were in our dorm room. Megan sat down and asked if, when we were allowed to move off campus, if I would want to live alone.

"We know you like to be alone, so we thought you might not mind it. And you're with Nick all the time so . . . " she said.

Taken aback, I felt like I might cry if I objected or said no. So my reaction was to appear strong, to show that I don't need anyone, my instinctual defense.

"Oh, yeah. That's okay. He'll probably be visiting a lot anyway," I replied with a fake smile.

This was the opposite of what my heart wanted, but I didn't know what else to say. I hoped that later we could go back and change this decision. I thought maybe I'd be able to gather my thoughts, think of what I would say, and ask if we could rethink it all. I thought that in a couple days we could talk about it again.

What I didn't know was that they'd already decided. Before even asking me, they'd signed a lease for an apartment without me. It was a done deal. I was so disconnected from them that they didn't even feel the need to ask me before signing the lease.

Since freshman year, I'd looked forward to living in our house with friends like my older sister had when she was in college, but now my exciting vision was gone. My friends were right—I did spend a lot of time alone or isolating with Nick.

The girl I once was—who had entered college living it up, always down for a good party with raspberry Smirnoff and orange Fanta—was gone. She was gone well before this living situation conversation. As my desire to be skinny grew, so did my desire to control my food intake. Alcohol scared me because I thought it would make me gain back all the weight I'd lost. That terrified me more than losing my friends, so I chose disordered eating over my friendships.

There was a part of me that truly didn't enjoy going out anymore, but I took it to an extreme. I was afraid of having even a drop of alcohol. My friends couldn't keep up. They didn't know who I was anymore, and neither did I. I never went out (I still don't love going out, hello movies on a Friday night), but I am authentically a fun person, with alcohol in my system dancing till three a.m. or no alcohol dancing until midnight. During my period of isolation and disordered eating, and despite my smaller body, I didn't have confidence that people would like me if I wasn't getting wasted all the time. I didn't think I would be accepted if I just went out without drinking or not staying out as late. I wasn't confident enough in any version of myself.

And it got worse. As I felt unloved by my friends, I disconnected from them even more. I was depressed and I didn't know where to turn. I felt further from my friends than ever before. Staying true to my need to appear strong,

I continued down the road to isolation, never once gaining the *true* strength to ask for help until over a year later. This went on until I broke up with Nick. That's when I could finally see that I needed my friends just as much as I needed a partner who loved me for me.

Let's talk about the healthy kind of friendships, the 90's sitcom sort of friendships. Yeah that's right, the admirable ones. Your tribe. Two things are important to note: number one, we must understand our own role in our friendships and learn how to appreciate and nurture them; number two, we must learn what to do when they aren't serving us in the positive ways we need.

Firstly, we must understand our own role in our friendships. When I was isolating from my friends, I still desperately yearned for love, belonging, and appreciation, but I was pushing it all away. I was sick. I needed to ask for help. Now looking back, I see how much of a major role I played. I pushed them away, I never voiced my struggles or leaned on them as I could have. That would have taken strength that I didn't have at the time. But had I leaned in, the doors to a much brighter reality would have opened for me. I was trying to recover from my disordered eating and hatred of myself *by* myself. That's like trying to tie your shoe with no hands, only your teeth. Unless you can do that, in which case, try using just your toes. That'll get ya.

When I am being my true, authentic self, my role in friendships is not to be the center of attention or the leader. I'm more reserved by nature, so I've always gravitated towards friendships in which I didn't feel the need to prove myself, be the loudest one there, or be the leader of the pack.

I'm thankful for that, but I don't think I've ever expressed to those friends how much it meant to me that they were and still are in my life. You have to appreciate and nurture your friendships. In high school, my Mom always told me, "You'd rather have one shiny quarter than one hundred dull pennies," meaning one quality friend is better than a bunch of friends you're not sure you can count on. I've always stuck to that.

Right now, I want you to take a step back. Take a good self-audit of how *you* are as a friend. Do you show your love and appreciation for them? Is it one-sided? Do you treat them as if they are a big shiny diamond that you cherish? How can you show that?

Buy them their favorite bath bomb and a facemask?

Give them a call, let them know you're thinking about them?

Pull a prank on them so you can laugh for hours and then thank them for always being there when you need a laugh?

Or, what about good old fashioned snail-mail? Write them a letter and actually mail it to them. Getting mail is so fun!

I'm the first to admit I don't do any of this enough. So along with you, friend, I am going to work on this as well. No one is perfect. All we can do is be intentional with the *most* important things in life and do our best to continue cultivating them.

Secondly, we need to look at the friendships that aren't serving us in the way we deserve.

As I worked hard to overcome my disordered eating by learning *true* nutrition and wellness, I also became aware that I was not alone in my struggles. Other people had unhealthy relationships with food and their bodies too, they just weren't working on it like I was. I would sit in the dining hall (during the period when I was working to overcome my struggles and heal . . . alone, of course) and see just how many other girls at my school were restricting. They would justify why they were eating something unhealthy, or not eating hardly anything on a Friday because they knew they were going to drink a substantial amount of calories that weekend.

I was stuck inside this culture. People didn't talk about any of it in a truly healthy, balanced way. It was normal to talk about the newest cleanse following spring break, or the extra hour on the treadmill after the weekend of binge drinking. Girls who wanted to lose weight before going on vacation would just stop eating carbs, or only eat salad, or go to extremes just like I did, some worse than others. Drinking more calories than you ate was common. These behaviors only caused more and more self-hatred for so many girls, like it had for me.

Again, I want you to get radically honest with yourself. Does your circle of friends fuel a desire to restrict? Does it fuel a desire to try a new fad diet because everyone else is? Does it fuel such a strong desire to be skinny that exercising comes before studying or work or relationships? Do you feel the need to be someone other than the person you truly are just to fit in? Do you feel drained and exhausted trying to be thinner or different because you don't feel you'd be loved and appreciated if you were just the real you?

There are certain relationships in our lives that are meant to teach us something. How might a friendship be teaching you to be strong and walk away? Or how might it be teaching you to be a leader and stand up for what you know is right (i.e., true health, true wellness, and healthy exercise)? How might it be teaching you to prioritize what is truly important right now? Could you spend those two extra hours studying, doing self-care, or parenting instead of at the gym, binging in the pantry, or drinking every night? Unhealthy relationships are always going to be available to us. We are in charge of which ones we nourish and which ones we allow to strengthen us.

Maybe you have friends who you've pushed so far away you don't know how to come back to them. Are they trying to help you but they just don't know how? Does your heart tell you that they are there for you, they love you as you are, and you don't need to be smaller or look a certain way to be loved?

We are not meant to find our best selves alone. We are meant to do it with people who fuel our fire for greatness. They are the ones who support you when you say you're going to create a sanctuary for lost pets or open a gymnasium for underprivileged children. They get just as excited as you and encourage you along the way. They are strong enough to offer their help when they notice you're going down a dangerous road. They model loving you when you're struggling to love yourself. Just like my relationship with Tyler, healthy romantic relationships model healthy friendships—they require a level of unending excitement and encouragement for each other's goals. This is a standard just as cheese on a pizza is standard.

But often, we don't choose these types of relationships or treat each other in this way. Judgment rages strong in our society. That darn Edna. We are quick to point fingers at others, with three pointing back at us. From wearing white in the winter, to how another mother parents her children, to a friend's decision to stay home instead of going out for the second night in a row. Just because another's decision is not that same as yours does not make it wrong. We pass judgment on others behind their backs, and many of us wouldn't dare say these things to their faces.

Everybody has a story. People change—sometimes for the better, sometimes for the worse. How often do we actually take a moment to step back and understand a person's sudden change? Going straight to judging Nancy for not being who she used to be by saying she's like a coke bottle shaken up and ready to explode at all times, constantly anxious, stressed, or on edge. We say things like, "She always says no when we ask to hang out, she's just different." Well, have you asked Nancy how she's doing, how you can help her, or if everything is okay? In the age of the most connection outlets, we are the most disconnected.

I encourage you to be the bigger person. Reach out when it seems like a friend in the group has changed or doesn't seem to be the same happy person they once were. *You* be the one who understands that everyone has a story, who understands that during difficult times all we need is a shoulder to lean on, someone to listen to our frustrations, and help us see the positive side in any situation. *I encourage you to be her.* And who wouldn't want to be the reason someone found their happiness again?

It means everything to have someone there for you when you're struggling. My story began with restriction, got more and more extreme, and then led me to an eventual turn to binge eating from my years of saying no to things I really loved. Emily was the one person I finally told that I was binge eating (see, I didn't find the courage to ask for help until deep into my experience with disordered eating) and she was the person that stuck with me through it all. She tried her best to help. Sometimes I didn't let her, but when the time came that I was finally strong enough to ask for help, I knew she was there. And she always will be.

On the same token, we need to forgive one another. The jealousy and competition that our subconscious brings about—gosh darn it, Helga—causes us to hurt the ones we love at times. Forgiveness is more for yourself than the other person. Forgiveness allows you to move past the difficult time to clear your own heart, but this time you can forgive and let go. When you know you have done everything in your power to make it great again but it can't be salvaged, then, sister, allow that person to go gracefully. They were a friend for a lesson in your life, not a lifetime.

We want strong and genuine friendships to round out our lady gang or man squad. Kind of like the wolf pack in the *Hangover*, minus all of the unfortunate events. How about we all make an agreement to get off of our phones, live for more than a highlight reel on social media, and cultivate human connection? Sounds like a great excuse to go get brunch with your lady gang if you ask me.

If you don't quite have a lady gang near you because you've moved, you're starting over, or you've decided to remove toxic relationships from your life, social media can be a wonderful thing for cultivating true community and connection. I was introduced to the Anywhere Office right after I moved to a state where the only person I knew was my sister. It's a community of like-minded young women who are passionate about changing the way the world views health and encouraging others to live a life of freedom and fulfillment. Also known as, my people. When you find your people, everything changes. Everything improves. It's like you have even more wonderful additions to your family. I like to think of it as God being like, "Shoot, forgot to make her your sister, so here's a non-biological sister." You feel even more loved, feel an even greater sense of community, and feel even more support. Less than one year later, I was hanging out in-person with some of the very best friends I have ever had, thanks to the Anywhere Office.

One spring, my friends from the Anywhere Office and I had a health and wellness conference in Phoenix, Arizona. We were sitting outside on the patio of the Airbnb after three full days of jam-packed learning and connecting with other wellness professionals, and we'd decided to spend the rest of the afternoon laying by the pool and playing piccolo all day into the night. We were a group of twelve girls, most of us having only met in person one time prior, some never at all. If there had been an outsider looking in, with the amount of laughter we had, they would've thought we'd been friends since kindergarten. The statement that we'd found our people is an understatement. To end the night, we sat around the table by the pool, sharing our goals for the next few years and what we wanted to accomplish together.

"I just have to say how grateful I am for you guys," Sarah said. "I don't talk much about it, but a couple of years ago my best friend passed away from cancer. I haven't felt true friendships since being with her, but I think I have finally found it with you all. You're the best friends I could ever ask for," she said.

We spent the next thirty minutes going around the table talking about how grateful we were for each other a bunch of happy crying messes. True connection is a gift from God. Best friends are siblings we were meant to have in our lives. Have faith. If you don't feel this great community and connection, your people are out there. Trust and have faith that you will find them. Start lookin', friend.

A little round up of the importance of loving friendships. This applies to you if:

- You have a friend struggling to love herself, going down a road you know is not meant for her
- You yourself have gone down a road you wish you hadn't and you need your friends back
- You want your current friendships to be stronger

1. Be the friend you want.

The power of visioning is so strong. I use it with my clients consistently and it never fails to be the thing that brings the most transformation and action. If you were to envision all of the qualities that made a truly incredible friend, what would they be? How would they act? What would they do?

Write down the top five qualities that make a true friend in your eyes.

_____

_____

_____

_____

_____

_____

In the next week, how can you embody one of those qualities? Each week, continue adding a quality until you fully embody that person yourself. Your lady gang will thank you.

2. Put yourself in her shoes.

Imagine you were struggling to find happiness and feel comfortable in your own skin, and you were heading down a road you knew was not good for you but you couldn't stop. What would you need from a friend? Practice patience and compassion. If you have a friend struggling with confidence issues, food or body image, or is acting in a way that is self-deprecating, know that she is experiencing a sort of trauma in her life. Trust me, she doesn't want to be going through it either. She's going to want to isolate and keep her distance. Be patient, always offer a helping hand, a shoulder to lean on, or just listen. Be a role model for her. If it is serious, always encourage her to ask for outside help. Just seeing that you truly care about her will soon be enough for her to gain the strength to ask for help.

If *you* are the one struggling, put yourself in your friends' shoes. How have you changed? Your friends may be confused, not able to understand what's happening. They miss you. Did you once trust them before? Trust them again and let them know that you are struggling. That, my dear, is true strength.

Take some time to reflect on who in your life you need to be a role model for, or where you've pushed great friends away. Take ten minutes and do what is called a "free write." This is where you write down absolutely everything that comes to mind, unedited. You may find relief in doing so, letting the words and thoughts get down on paper instead of having to carry them in your head or heart.

_____

_____

_____

_____

_____

3. Call your own crap.

Be the bigger person. Acknowledge the wrongdoings you've committed. Recognize where you've placed unfair judgment. This will be one of the most powerful practices you can bring into the rest of your life. Someone who is able to call themselves out on their own wrongdoings is someone who also demands respect in return.

4. The F word, again.

I know we've talked about this a lot already, but you've got to forgive again.

Get used to being the bigger person and making forgiveness a habit. Friendships will not always last, and just the simple act of forgiving may not repair what was broken. But for your own sake in not having to carry the burden any longer, forgive. Hopefully the friendship is strong and this will only make it stronger. If it does, you, sister, have one of those shiny quarters and a friendship that will last a lifetime.

Write down every person you need to forgive, whether it be in person, over the phone, or through prayer. Forgive them all one by one, including yourself.

_____

_____

_____

_____

_____

Friendships are special. They make life fun and exciting. They make life easier, and it's worth fighting for your life-giving friendships. You deserve the best, now you just have to allow yourself to have it. What would the best version of you do?

CHAPTER 5

When a treadmill minute equals beach-day minute, you know you've made it.

"Fitness isn't about being better than someone else. It's about being better than you used to be."

—An overused quote on Pinterest that speaks to my soul by a man named anonymous.

I T WAS JUST after we started officially dating (finally), and T had moved back to Colorado after a couple weeks of summer at home in Michigan. We were two weeks into my three-week stay with him in Colorado. We both love adventures, big and small, so naturally, every weekend and many of our weekdays we went on at least one adventure. You guessed it, since we were in Colorado this usually included hiking boots and a mountain trail of some sort.

We were at Estes Park in Rocky Mountain National park for one particular adventure, getting ready to hike up to the very top of Sky Pond. If you've never heard of Sky Pond, well, this is the one and only time I'm going to tell you that you need to take a break from reading and put this book down ASAP. Yep, put it down and google "Sky Pond."

Gorgeous right?

I'm not sure if you saw the hike description, but it is recorded as a "strenuous" nine-mile hike. We went all out for this one. We got a hotel close to the trailhead, woke up early to beat the rush so we could get to the top and enjoy the "strenuous" climb before the crowds rushed in. We brought some snacks to help us through and wore all the layers to prepare for the chilly top even though it was only September.

About thirty minutes into the hike, I looked around and noticed that the mountain top seemed to be getting smaller instead of bigger. This was a given sign that it was getting further away, even to a newbie hiker like me. "Hmm, that doesn't seem right," I thought.

"Wait, let's make sure we're on the right trailhead," Tyler said. He pulled out his iPhone to google it and, well, no service. It was like the rainbow wheel of death, but worse. We continued on, Tyler saying this was probably right.

An elderly couple passed us, "Wow, I want to be like them when we're older. Hiking a trail like this at their age, that's amazing!" I said.

A little while later, another elderly couple passed us. This time, they seemed a tad less in shape if you're picking up what I'm laying down. Another passed, and another. About an hour into the hike, the mountain top seemingly much farther away than before. I said, "Are you sure this is right?"

Hey, I trusted him. He had four years at the Air Force Academy, multiple survival trainings and was actually the instructor for the younger cadets' survival training. *And,* he'd done this hike before. But beginning to question my judgment in trusting his navigation skills, I said, "No really, I think we should ask someone," to which he smiled and agreed as the tenth old couple passed us, having seen no young and energetic individuals like ourselves yet.

Friends. My lovely, incredibly intelligent (except for his navigation skills) hubby-to-be led me FOUR MILES IN THE WRONG DIRECTION. Not one, not two. *Four miles.* I'm laughing just thinking about it. Four miles in the wrong direction, meaning we'd have to go another four miles to get back to the beginning and restart our nine-mile *strenuous* hike. Do the math. Four miles each way, back to the beginning, then nine, plus walking to and from the parking lot. Mama had full reason to be royally peeved, enraged, hopping mad, in a tizzy. But friends, I laughed until my stomach hurt. This is one of those stories he will never live down. Especially now that I put it in a published book. Sorry, babe.

We went the four miles back and began our hike from the true beginning, turning right instead of left, heading to the top of the mountain instead of the bottom this time. Despite the painfully long detour, it was one of the most breathtaking days of my life. The views were incomparable. Excuse my cheesy self, but I felt the presence of God's creation with us all day. What a blessing that we were able to complete a strenuous hike, which sweet Tyler made even strenuous-er. We got to see lakes, animals, mountain sides, and waterfalls we'd never have been able to see if not on foot. That day, I thanked God for the many blessings I had. My able-body, my conditioned heart and lungs, my strong legs, my loving heart, and that dear tenth old couple showing us our (Tyler's) four-mile mistake.

Our bodies are so strong and capable, especially when we feed and condition them adequately. If I hadn't been a lover of fitness, I might not have been able to complete that hike. I might not have been able to climb the waterfall to finally reach the top. I might not have been able to climb the rock wall to finally see Sky Pond, no matter how much of a newbie I looked like in the process. I might not have ever seen the indescribable views as we sat at the very top of Sky Pond, overlooking what seemed like the world. Feeling completely at peace, serene, and thankful. Maybe I would have completed it, but as a whiny girlfriend, or completely in pain and immobile for days following.

Exercise truly is a blessing, not a chore. I know, I know. You're rolling your eyes because you've heard that numerous times before, but we have an obligation to love our bodies so that we see it as such. Think about it–swimming in beautiful lakes or seas, hiking extraordinary mountains, skiing down beautiful slopes, or running lakeside trails are some of life's greatest adventures. Having the ability to condition our bodies to experience memories such as these is a gift.

Exercise is not something we need to use to fuel an inner-hate for our bodies. Doing an extra hour on a cardio machine to cancel out our food isn't treating your body with the love and respect it deserves. We can be just as unhealthy in the form of weak and exhausted by abusing exercise in the same way never exercising at all is unhealthy.

I began this chapter about exercise this way for a reason. I didn't begin by talking about running, or lifting, or Crossfit, or any of that. That's because the type of exercise you choose really doesn't matter. It's not about doing what's "hot," or what's new, or what's going to give you the fastest or best results. It's the fact that having a healthy and able-body is a gift many individuals don't get. Whether it be a debilitating injury, birth defect, or something of that nature, we often forget exercise is something we *get to do*.

Movement, working out, exercising or whatever you want to call it is a critical piece in creating the health and confidence of your dreams, but also the life of your dreams. Let's step away from the idea that exercise creates the "body figure" you want for a moment. It can, there's a time and place for those types of exercise talks, and we'll get to that, but that all means nothing if we don't first establish the importance of a healthy approach to fitness.

This is where I know my opinion differs from others in my industry, so stick with me here. There comes a point when our bodies keep us from living our best life and being our best selves. If you're so full of junk food, weak from little to no movement, or out of shape that you can no longer walk up a flight of stairs comfortably or go for a brisk walk with your loved ones, then we have to take a step back. Maybe you're consistently exhausted from overdoing exercise, not eating enough, and you hardly have the stamina to live life outside of fitness. We must seek balance, regardless of where you fall on the spectrum.

If you're so uncomfortable in your own skin that you refuse to go to the beach or participate in certain activities, then we have to have a chat with your inner highest self, and I mean that in the most loving way possible. We need to love ourselves inside our own body at every single stage, one hundred and fifty million percent. That will never change from being my number one step.

Exercise has so many benefits besides aesthetic ones such as:

- Reduces risk for disease such as diabetes, heart disease, and other chronic illnesses
- Promotes better sleep
- Improves your mood by releasing endorphins
- Increases your energy
- Supports brain health and memory
- Increases confidence

One of my favorite benefits of exercise is being able to connect with like-minded people and find friendships with similar interests. It's a way to connect with your friends and loved ones. Although, if you decide to go on a hike together, I do suggest bringing a map.

Imagine yourself in a consistently better mood, finding daily happiness, having more energy to study, work, or play. Imagine yourself not getting sick quite as often, sleeping more deeply, and having more confidence. When you envision your best self, the person you are trying to be, does she have most of these things? I'm guessing the answer is yes! "If you want to deliver value in this world, it's all about treating oneself first. When you treat yourself first and you create the perfect vessel, you then have the ability to affect so many more globally[8]." When you treat your body right, you fill your own cup, and you feel the absolute best you've felt in your life, that is when you will truly begin to leave lasting value to those around you.

Yet in Edna's world today, we tend to think of exercise purely as something that makes you lose weight. You have to do a certain type to achieve a certain body. Grit through the pain, keep pushing, and even if you hate it, you should just keep doing it. This is how I viewed the fitness world when I began my road to losing the weight I'd put on freshman year. I am very blessed to have never really "abused" exercise to the extent that so many unfortunately do (i.e., hours upon hours of exercise or using it to negate what was just eaten). I truly did love it and wanted to do it consistently because of that, but I fell into the trap of feeling like I *had* to do certain types of exercise in order to achieve the body I wanted.

Before becoming so obsessed with getting a six pack or the best body I could have, I loved running, lifting, and high intensity interval (HIIT) workouts. I still do. One of the things I looked forward to were my long distance runs every

---

8 The School of Greatness: A Real-World Guide to Living Bigger, Loving Deeper, and Leaving a Legacy.

Saturday morning. The endorphin rush, mental clarity, and sense of peace that blanketed me through running brought me to a blissful state. I lifted and did HIIT during the week and ran on the weekends, sometimes during the week as well.

But then I decided I wanted abs. What did the gurus say about running and having a strong fit body? Do less cardio. I had a very addictive personality, even today it's something I have to be aware of to not go too far. When I decided to do something, I went all in, often to an unhealthy extent. So by hearing that I should do less cardio, I said bye bye to my weekend runs. I didn't see it as a negative thing because I did (and do) love lifting so much. I thought, "I am just tailoring my fitness program toward my goals." At first glance, this wasn't an issue and wouldn't have ever been an issue if I didn't deny myself of what I truly wanted.

What I truly wanted, what my heart was begging me for, was to go for a long run. My gut was pleading to just let my legs run free along the waterside, take in the beauty of the morning, and let my mind be at ease. But I ignored those pleas because my mind said, "That will take away from the muscle you've built. You'll regress and all the hard work you've put in to build muscle will go to waste." It took me years after I'd healed my relationship with food and cultivated a strong sense of self-love that I even realized what I was doing. It was to the point that if I was following a fitness plan and a friend wanted to go workout together, I would do my fitness plan workout beforehand to be sure I followed it as precisely as possible, then later go workout with her. Different forms of exercise didn't feel like options for me, not because I didn't think they sounded fun, but because I was so preoccupied with the "best and fastest" method to the body I wanted. Does this sound familiar? Read on.

I have a really good friend, Justine, who is also a health coach focused on balanced eating and exercise. Justine came into the fitness industry with an obsession with getting the "perfect body," similar to my story. She went even further down this road and competed in numerous figure competitions. If you're not familiar with what a figure competition is, it is a sport where you are judged by your physique, often getting unhealthily lean for the day of the competition.

From the outside, Justine appeared to be living the dream. She had the body, she was approached with numerous endorsement contracts, and had a consistent personal training career. What the outside couldn't see, however, was that she was abusing her body, felt truly miserable, and suffered from debilitating anxiety, all for a certain body. This caused her to hate exercise. She didn't look forward to going and equated it with having to look a certain way. Eventually in 2014, she was abruptly confronted with her unhealthy reality. Forced to step away from competing and fitness modeling from adrenal fatigue and thyroid dysfunction (an effect of not fueling the body properly and over exercising), she decided this way of viewing food and exercise just wasn't worth it.

The following year, she put the pieces of her happiness back together. One foot in front of the other, she discovered a balance of the less-than-nutritious foods she loved with the nutritious foods that made her feel her best—a kale salad with a beer, if you will. Her passion to spread the word of balanced nutrition and exercise to propel others into their happiest life has now become her career. Her company name is the cutest: "Crunches then Cocktails." Isn't that the best? She's fallen in love with cycling and pure barre, two forms of exercise she never would have done if a friend didn't encourage her to try them.

What do these stories mean? They mean that exercise is about more than shaping a body you desire. It's a method of cultivating deeper self-love and appreciation. It's to be used for stress relief, to gain more happiness, to find a better mood, to gain more energy, to find some "me time," and as an addition to an even higher quality of life. As with all things, there are two sides to the spectrum. Maybe you keep on the side of never exercising, insisting you hate it yet feeling guilty for never going, or maybe you exercise for hours at a time. You deny yourself of healthy rest and recovery until you get the "perfect body," or you add an extra hour of cardio after a night out, a side effect of guilt. Whichever side of the spectrum you find yourself on, know that finding your balanced middle will allow you to live your best life and become the best version of you that you could ever imagine. Having the time and mental capacity to focus on what's important, to be in the moment, to finally live in a body you feel proud and confident in—it is possible and it's more than worth it. It's what you deserve.

So how do you know how much exercise, what kind, and how often? Remember when I suggested that my point of view was a bit different than others in my industry? I do think exercise on top of a healthy eating regimen is necessary to get to the point of being your best self. If you "hate" exercise and never do it, I say you're wrong. You just haven't found one you love. If you "can't" get yourself to wake up early to go, or to go after work because your mind is screaming for the couch, quit your excuses. It truly means you haven't found *your* method of exercise yet. There *is* an exercise regimen you can love, that brings you the energy and mood benefits you want, a routine you can do out of habit even if you're not in the mood. You just haven't found it yet or haven't stood up to your mind's messages from Helga (that pesky subconscious that is saying you hate exercise) and made it into a newfound love. I'm a little bit of tough love coupled with your biggest cheerleader on this topic. Like a teddy bear that means business.

If you google search "the best workout," what you'll find is a lot of different people trying to convince you that their method is the best method. The truth is that the body needs and benefits from a combination of all types of exercise, i.e., strength training, cardiovascular training, and flexibility. Remember, my goal in this book is to help *you* become the very best, most confident, happiest version of *you*. In reading this, keep in mind that the number one goal is to make sure you're loving what you're doing.

A quick little overview of each:

Strength training is loosely defined as "a method of improving muscular strength by gradually increasing the ability to resist force to stimulate muscle strength through the use of free weights, machines, or the person's own body weight[9]."

---

9 The Free Dictionary. (medical-dictionary.thefreedictionary. com).

Examples of strength training include:

- Traditional weight training
- CrossFit
- Pure Barre
- Pilates

Cardiovascular training is loosely defined as "an activity continually maintained and performed rhythmically . . . used to stimulate and challenge your muscles, heart, and lungs[10]." There are two forms of cardio I believe are most important to explain in order to help you keep your body strong and in the best condition. These are low intensity steady state cardio (LISS) and high intensity interval training (HIIT). If you are without prior injury or risk, performing a mix of both types in your routine is most beneficial. LISS is loosely explained by "keeping your intensity low (approximately 65%) for long periods of time your body is encouraged to use fat stores[11]."

Examples of LISS include:

- Jogging
- Walking

---

10 Heeter, Kris, "The ACSM Definition of Cardiovascular Exercise," AZ Central, (https://healthyliving.azcentral.com/acsm-definition-cardiovascular-exercise-18723.html)

11 (http://fitnessorstrength.com/fitness/what-is-liss-cardio/)

- Swimming
- Biking

On the other hand, HIIT is loosely explained by periods of working out in which an all-out effort is given, followed by short periods of rest or active recovery and then repeated for a certain amount of time. Because of the consistent elevated heart rate, this type of training burns more calories in less time. "A high-intensity workout increases the body's need for oxygen during the effort and creates an oxygen shortage, causing your body to ask for more oxygen during recovery[12]." This creates the EPOC effect (excess post exercise oxygen consumption) which causes the body to burn more calories for up to thirty-six hours post exercise.

Examples of HIIT include:

- Sprints (running, biking, stair stepper, etc.)
- Every minute on the minute (EMOM)
- As many rounds as possible (AMRAP)
- Tabata—twenty seconds of work, ten seconds of rest for eight rounds, a total of four minutes

For obvious reasons, HIIT is a very popular form of exercise for its fat loss benefits. However, performing this type of exercise too often can cause an increase in the amount of cortisol production which is the stress hormone.

---

12 "The Do-It-Anywhere HIIT Workout You Need to Try," Daily Burn.

Overproduction of cortisol signals fat production as a defense mechanism from physiological stress, making losing fat even harder to accomplish. Along with increased cortisol production, too much intense exercise without proper rest and recovery can cause poor immunity, injury, irritability, and more harmful effects.

When it comes to working out, I'm all about smarter, not harder. If you're excuse is "I don't have time," well sister, you wrong. All of my workouts are under an hour. The best way to keep it short is to be sure your heart rate is elevated consistently. HIIT is one of my favorite ways to train because it is quick and efficient, and the endorphin rush makes me feel like I'm a puppy that just got a new chew toy. I like to incorporate it into my schedule one to four times per week. Not only is it quick and effective, but it's a great way to combine cardio training with resistance training if done with EMOM, AMRAP, or Tabata.

Lastly, rest and recovery are key to an optimal physical body. We build muscle when we're resting. Healthy stress response is maintained by proper frequency, not over-doing it. You can achieve mental and physical optimization through consistency, so be sure to end your workouts with a good stretch, end your evening with a foam rolling session, or begin your day with gentle stretching or yoga as well. And sister, get those Z's at night, at least seven to nine hours!

I'm not going to go too far into detail because this basic knowledge and information is all you need. On top of that, pick a variation from each category (strength, cardio, and flexibility) that you look forward to doing.

Friends. I know yoga is so good for me, but I'm like

bambi on ice when I go. I'm just not good at it and most of the time I don't enjoy it. If you love to get your Namaste on, then girl, YES. Fill that schedule up with yoga classes alongside your running days. I'm more of the type that blasts Eminem in my headphones for a good lift and Tabata session instead. If it doesn't feel like I'm in the club about to get my twerk on, then it's just not right! Sister, my point is to find what you love, own it, and make it a habit.

Developing a consistent workout schedule you love, where you know you're going to go consistently and quit being a lazy bum, is an important point to make. On the opposite side of the spectrum, many of us workout because we think it cancels out what we ate. A pizza the night before, a late-night snack after drinking, or having "too many _____" seems to be reason for us to need to work out an extra hour. Maybe we don't take a rest day because we don't think we "earned" it—this is just as unhealthy as not working out at all. This is just as bad for your body as being a couch potato. Your body needs rest. Over-exercise can lead to adrenal fatigue, a weakened immune system, and many other negative effects, not to mention an unhealthy mindset and appreciation for yourself.

I encourage you to again step back and examine your mentality when it comes to movement and exercise. What is your motivation? Why do you choose to go? How do you choose what types? If your answers to these questions are along the lines of "I love it," "it is my me-time," "it is my greatest stress reliever," "It's my favorite way to catch up with friends," then you do you, boo.

If the answers to these questions are more like, "I had too

many sweets yesterday," "I hate the way I look," "I still don't love the skin I'm in," then you deserve more. You deserve better. It's not about the exercise, it's not about the way you look or the number on the scale. It's about being the person *you were created* to be. We can't be the best mother, friend, employee, or fill in the blank if we're exhausted trying to combat every calorie eaten. Reframe your mindset, find love for yourself at every stage, and then gaining confidence and pride in your body will come naturally. The binging will subside. The restriction will be no longer. Hold tight for some journaling prompts to help you make these mindset shifts at the end of the chapter.

Again, I know this probably isn't the first time you're hearing these things, but how many times are you going to have to hear them until you understand this is the most important step to take? How long is it going to take for you to understand that the happiness, love for your body, confidence, or any other goal will not come until you understand *true health* and balance mind, body, and soul? Let me be the voice you need to help you understand that no amount of knowledge, "best body formula," or dieting will bring you to the body you want, the confidence you want, or the happiness you want until you decide that you deserve more. Have the appreciation for yourself to get off the couch if you never exercise. Have the love for yourself to rest if you know your body is overworked from too much exercise. Have the strength to create your version of balance to truly be the healthiest version of you.

Now that you understand rule number one we can discuss an appropriate plan.

1. Get your mind right.

If your mindset around movement and exercise is not healthy, your body and your life cannot be healthy either. A healthy and thriving body means having a healthy and thriving career, relationships, social life—everything.

You may either be an under-exerciser or an over-exerciser. Wherever you find yourself, consider the following journaling prompts to move you from stuck to thriving.

Close your eyes, settle into your seat, and imagine the very best version of you. She's happy, peaceful, in love with every day, healthy in her relationships, being the healthiest version of herself, thriving in a career she loves—fill in the blanks.

When you imagine this highest version of yourself, what is her mindset when it comes to exercise?

How does she exercise? How often? What types?

What are the thoughts she thinks about herself? About exercise? About a balanced healthy lifestyle?

_____

_____

_____

_____

_____

Starting right now, what is one thing that you can do to be the highest version of yourself? Perhaps it's journaling daily to remind yourself of the person you are trying to become. Maybe it's catching yourself every time you look in the mirror and see flaws instead of beauty. Or maybe it's choosing to stick to an exercise routine for the first time. Pick one thing and make it your number one focus for the next week. Make it your number one until it's a normal thing for you, and you're one step closer to truly being that version of yourslef. Then pick another, and another. This is not overnight. Don't put a time limit on it. Focus on creating this mental shift until you feel your rigidity loosen, or your lack of motivation subside.

2. Find your exercise plan.

When finding an exercise program that works for you, I always look at goals first. What is your goal? To run a half marathon? To feel strong as heck? To just feel good in your own skin? All of these goals would have a different training program according to the outcome you're looking for.

To feel strong as heck, look for a strength-based fitness plan with a healthy amount of cardio. It's my favorite way to train and I love the mentality it gives me. I encourage all women to give strength training a try if they haven't. Oh, and I'm sure you've heard this a few times too, but I'll be the voice you need to hear to believe it. Strength training does not make you bulky. Gaining muscle burns the fat in its place and achieves the "toned" look we so often strive for.

To run a half marathon, you might run most days of the week and incorporate cross training (i.e. biking, strength, or recovery) for the proper strength and endurance.

To feel your very best in your own skin, your routine can truly be anything. Pure barre mixed with lifting and spinning? Running mixed with flexibility and strength-focused yoga? Try it all out! Have fun with it. See what makes you excited to hop out of bed in the morning or feel like Beyoncé on stage walking out of the gym.

It's not one-size-fits-all and it gets to be what you want it to be. For specific goals like a half marathon and such, look for a trainer you trust and love and dive into the programs they offer. There are numerous online trainers these days with very low priced and often free program options. Start there!

3. Make sure you love it

I think we all know by now how important this is, so I contemplated not even making this a step. But just so you thoroughly understand and act on it this time, you've got to love it like Kanye loves Kanye.

This will ensure that you do it consistently, even on the days you don't feel like it, but know that you'll feel your best when you do. It'll turn into a habit and your new health regimen will truly be a healthy *lifestyle*.

Loving it also ensures your mental health is strong. When you go because you truly want to, then we can be sure you're going for the right reasons. Your mindset will be more positive on difficult days, you'll find stress-relief in the healthiest form, and you might even meet new friends with similar interests in the process.

To assess your love for your current training program, consider your answers to the following questions:

What is my motivation for my current exercise program (or lack thereof)? For example, because you think you need to? Because it's what so-and-so does and you want legs like hers? Because you feel like you eat too much, or your stomach is too fluffy? You just don't like working out—you're not one of those people? You get the picture.

Take a step back and truly do a self-audit. Remember step one and imagine the absolute best version of yourself.

_____

_____

_____

_____

4. Schedule it in.

To help my clients begin working out if they aren't into the habit quite yet, I give them the trick to schedule it in as if it were a doctor's appointment. Would you cancel on your doctor? Hopefully not! Every Sunday take a look at your schedule and write down the days and times you are going to get some movement in. You could take it a step further and create accountability with a friend. Then stick to it like it's the greatest promise you've ever made yourself. It just might be.

If those excuses roll up again, for example, "I don't have time," "It's not as important as _____," or what have you, remember the promise you've made to yourself. Remember *why* you want to be the healthiest version of you. These excuses could swing in the opposite direction as well. For example, "I need to go an extra hour because I ate too much last night," and so on. That is not healthy either. That is not being the healthiest version of yourself. Determine a healthy amount of exercise to do each week and stick to that.

5. Monthly check-in.

Every month or so, take a look at your current routine. Answer the following questions:

Does this routine keep me challenged?

Do I enjoy this routine?

What is my mindset after a workout in this routine?

Consistently re-evaluate to keep yourself progressing, in a healthy mindset, and keeping things fresh and exciting!

And there it is. That's it. We don't have to make it difficult. If you haven't caught the gist yet, it's about connecting with the highest version of you, and acting as if you already are her today. Loving yourself through the process. Doing it because you love it and putting in the effort to discover what you truly do love, and feeling like a pop star with a glittery concert outfit on every time you walk out of that workout session.

CHAPTER 6

How to hate kale and still be healthy

"I'll take a kale salad with an extra spoonful of magic seeds and plant-based dirt dressing on the side, with a dairy-free, sugar-free, gluten-free, vegan, extra protein cupcake without the cake and extra unicorn sprinkles please."

—Say that ten times fast.

Do you want to know the very best way to eat for a body you're confident in? We're talking about major secrets here. The quickest, fastest, surefire way to the body you are so stinking proud of? No? Oh, okay. Shoot, I had a whole chapter on it.

Just kidding, the chapter is here. Do you want to know? Alright, here you have it: skinny teas, fat-loss pills, and waist belts.

Jokes. No, it's not those things. Can you tell I'm fluent in sarcasm?

Don't worry, I once believed in these things too. I've bought "skinny tea." I've tried fat loss pills and almost everything else. None of it ever worked for achieving true health or the body I so desperately wanted. If you read the fine print on most of those things what you see is, "For best results must be accompanied by proper nutrition and exercise." Also known as, it doesn't work but proper nutrition and exercise does.

So many of us are willing to spend hundreds, sometimes even thousands, on weight loss supplements for the twisted peace of mind that we might actually be successful *this* time. But hardly any of us is willing to put forth continuous effort or invest in a program where we can learn the proper tools to not only find a healthy weight on our own, but learn to make it something we can actually see ourselves doing for an extended period of time. We might go all in for a few weeks, but quickly lose hope and fall back into old patterns. We so often choose the drastic program that promises "results fast," without regard to whether we actually find pleasure in following through on that program, let alone be able to sustain it. We invest more in outside resources that aren't guaranteed to work in order to cover up the fact that we don't actually believe in ourselves enough to make it happen in the healthiest way, on our own. Scary, right?

This is because of a few things: number one, we have a tendency to make proper nutrition really freakin' complicated; and number two, its written into our patterning. Helga gets to take the blame for that one.

First, we make it so damn hard. Take the quote at the beginning of this chapter for instance. It may seem like I'm poking fun at those who do choose to be vegan, gluten free, or what have you, but that's not the case. I myself am dairy-free, mostly refined sugar-free, and only include high-quality grains into my diet most of the time. I have reasoning for it *and* a very healthy relationship with food. Read on to see why. My point is that most of the time, we over-complicate it. Most believe that healthy eating is confusing, lacking in flavor, boring, expensive, time consuming, or a combination of these attributes. I'm here to tell you that healthy eating can and will be delicious and even easy for you, if you follow the simple tips and guidelines I will show you in this chapter.

At ten years old, a few weeks after I was diagnosed with insulin resistance syndrome, my family was doing everything they could to support me. We took all candy out of the house, bought wheat bread instead of white, started cooking healthier, and asked the servers for special accommodations to help manage my insulin resistance syndrome. One day, my mom was explaining to my aunt and uncle what we were doing to help me get on the right track. My uncle's advice?

"If it tastes good, spit it out." Oh, my word, is that so wrong.

But this is just what he'd learned over the course of his life. During most of his young life and present adulthood, much of the nutrition media spoke about how in order to be healthy, one must be low-carb, low-fat, sugar-free, along with a lot of other garbage rules.

Thank the Lordy we now have up-to-date research and findings proving that this isn't necessarily true.

When we're looking to make the switch into healthier habits, going head first into the nutrition world can be daunting. There are a lot of foods out there that are incredibly nutritious, but also just beginning to make their way into everyday vocabulary and making it seem like healthy food needs to be from another planet. Take spirulina, for instance. It sounds like a children's book character if you ask me, but it's actually a highly nutritious type of algae containing high amounts of nutrients, and it's also a complete protein. Regardless, it is understandable why one might be confused or discouraged just hearing the name.

Even if you're not a newbie to the health world, it can all be utterly confusing. My advice? Make it simple. One day at a time. One step at a time. One new habit at a time. Acquire a basic understanding you can manage and feel confident in. That's what I'm here to show you how to do.

We all know by now that I have tried it all. Eliminating different foods (because the gurus told me I had to), only eating "clean," meal-timing, and on and on it goes. What I've found through my own experience and years of training is that all of that is just minutia. It's easy to think that to be successful, we have to do it all, follow it to a T, include all of those little details, and be perfect in order to be successful in the timeframe we want. That is not the case.

I'm going to show you what you *do* need to know and follow through on. But first, we must dive more deeply into the way you view food. After that short period of too many (okay, maybe like eight months' worth) raspberry Smirnoff and orange Fanta drinks helped me gain a few pounds (okay, more than a few), my mind was set on the idea of just losing that weight and getting back to where I was before. I went into it with the focus of getting the weight off rather than improving my overall wellbeing. It did not seem possible that I could feel better about myself as a person along my journey to losing the weight or even appreciate my body. In my mind, food was something to be controlled in order to lose weight. I had the basic understanding of nutritious versus not nutritious (Reese's no, broccoli yes), but not enough to know how to lose weight in a healthy manner or create balanced, nutritious meals aside from simply eating less.

So, I went head first into dieting. I tried to eat as clean and "flat belly friendly" as possible. I cut many things (regardless of nutrient density) out of my diet because the self-proclaimed gurus said I had to. I meticulously tracked my intake and timed every meal for many years. I unknowingly created a major disconnect with my body's hunger and fullness signals and fear of different foods, the biggest being alcohol. Today, I'm not a huge drinker—I just don't enjoy the feeling of it—but there is a *major* difference between not wanting to drink because you're afraid of gaining weight and not wanting to drink because you just don't want to.

All of this restriction caused me to lose touch with my body's hunger cues. I no longer listened to my body when it cried for nourishment or didn't feel hungry, because my plan said to eat every three hours, so that's what I did. I ate how much my food tracking app told me to eat regardless of whether I was full or hungry. I couldn't tell if my mind was hungry or if my stomach truly was. I didn't trust that my body knew how to tell me what I needed and when. I couldn't differentiate between which foods actually made me feel good and which did not. I also didn't trust that I could make progress toward a stronger, more fit body if I wasn't meticulously tracking everything. The ideal body felt more important than my peace of mind, and I thought I wouldn't have the happiness or peace of mind *until* I had the body.

One night, well after I'd lost the weight I'd put on freshman year, I was laying in my bed in my dorm room for my nightly routine of inputting my meals into my tracking app for the next day. After trying a few different combinations of meal ideas, I finally had it all perfectly in my food tracking app for the macro numbers I had calculated online for the fastest way to the goal body I needed. The next day, I woke up excited to make progress, but by the end of that day when I went to have dinner, it didn't quite sound appetizing anymore. What *did* sound appetizing didn't "fit my macros." It was off by 5-10 grams and to me, that was appalling.

I was in a daily internal battle, no matter how much I wanted to avoid it. I'd be at mental war with myself for either eating foods that sounded appetizing, or the meal I'd already logged that fit my macros perfectly. Quite frankly, that meal I craved more would still have had me "on the right track," but I was obsessed with my plan and perfection, unwilling to do anything that wouldn't give me my goal body as quickly as possible.

Tracking was mentally unhealthy for me at that time because I wanted perfection. I wanted results quickly. I was desperate to have the dream body. I needed to be perfect until I'd reached my goal. You know the story—I would reach my goals but I was never satisfied, always wanting to see more muscles. I'd never let myself have a meal that just sounded delicious. Get this, I'd never let myself have it even if it really *was* healthy and nutritious. I was addicted to controlling my food. My focus was on results, perfect numbers, and my body's appearance. But what I found unacceptable in my body, others didn't even notice. Rather, others found my body to be *their* goal body, but I never allowed myself to see what they saw. My mentally-healthy freshman-year-self wouldn't have believed I'd ever get that obsessed and disconnected from my true self.

My focus should have been on understanding what I secretly thought that "better body" would bring me: more confidence, stronger relationships, love and appreciation for *myself,* daily happiness and positivity, and feeling like I had my s**t together. If I had known what I was truly looking for, I could have made healthy action steps and understood how to find flexibility and freedom in a healthy lifestyle. Then, I could have reached the true goals I had set.

Looking back at this now, if someone had shown me that finding an understanding of what food could do *for* me, it would have helped me reach my goal in a much (much much much, much much MUCH much) healthier way. At that time, I didn't believe I had the "body type" to be able to do it in the more balanced way people spoke of. News flash, Helga taught me that and it's not true, not for me or you. I could have bypassed the disordered eating and found a much happier version of me much faster. If you had a dollar every time I said "much," huh?

That is why I'm digging into our subconscious before we get to the breakdown of nutrition. Most of us have food habits that are written into our patterning, which Helga holds onto like a baby holds a security blanket. This means we created habits around food when we were young children, most likely given to us by our parents or parental figures, which have stayed with us into adulthood.

Take a look at where you stand at this moment. Not literally—actually, if you're standing you should probably sit down while you're reading. What is your current "starting point" for finding your version of a healthy, balanced lifestyle? Do you need to reign in the Oreos? Are you looking to have more energy, get sick less often, eat a few more green things? Or do you need to find balance in the other direction, and allow yourself some less than nutritious things every now and then? Some of you may be addicted to fast food with a risk for illness, and some of you may be under-eating, developing fears of foods or never allowing yourself to be "less clean." Or maybe you're somewhere in the middle. The truth is, most people can improve their nutrition in some way. Regardless of where you land on the spectrum, it will be most beneficial to observe your habits and identify your triggers. Ask yourself:

- What causes you to eat less than nutritious foods more often than you'd like?

- What causes you to disregard your earlier commitment to more veggies and opt for dessert instead?

- What causes you to not allow yourself to have the burrito you've been craving and get the salad instead even though your mind is craving balance?

- What causes you to over-indulge at night?

I've had quite a few clients who used food to cope with stress. One in particular told me, "I know the impulse comes at night when I sit down to watch TV. I see it coming but it gets to a point where my body is just on auto-pilot and I can't stop. Diana, I feel like I black out and lose control of my own mind. I desperately want to stop, but it's as if I'm a robot who's stuck on 'eat to numb out' mode."

Many people find comfort in food after a stressful day. Many people numb out after a fight with loved ones with a pint of Ben and Jerry's. Other people just feel lonely and soothe themselves with food. Maybe you were told during your childhood that you weren't pretty enough, so salad is all you get. Maybe you started dieting at a very young age, and food restriction is all you know, or maybe food has always been your reward for a job well done.

Where did these habits begin? Why? At one point in your life, either using food for comfort or manipulating it was your mind's best solution to try to keep you happy. These patterns literally get chemically wired into our brains making it difficult to change, but it doesn't have to end there. It just so happens that you're ready for an upgrade. You know better now, so now you get to do better. You get to rewire your mind. You get to find a healthy balance. You get to find happiness and confidence in your own skin.

If you find yourself troubled with these habits, have no fear, Diana is here. Dear Lord, I'm too much sometimes. In the next chapter, we'll dive a bit deeper into the habit side of food and how to replace your unhealthy habits with better ones. But going over this first gives me peace of mind that you'll be strong enough to be honest with yourself then and begin eating healthier in a balanced way, for the right reasons.

Now, the moment we've all been waiting for. What really makes a food nutritious? How can you create balanced meals so that you can truly eat everything you want and *still* be making progress toward your most confident body? How can you find your version of balance with food? To have the ability to create a balanced meal and feel in charge of your nutritional health, a basic and proper understanding of nutrition is necessary.

First, start your day with an organic, non-GMO, star fruit, kale, parsley, plants-grown-in-the-holy-land smoothie blended with holy water instead of juice.

I'm totally kidding, but I do love smoothies and I kind of feel bad I just joked about them. First, let's talk nutrients, macro and micro. These are the avocado to your toast in the balanced nutrition world.

Macronutrients consist of proteins, fats, and carbohydrates, each of which your body needs in large amounts. Each plays a key role in your body's energy levels, efficiency, composition, and so much more. Quite literally, food is our fuel.

Micronutrients are vitamins and minerals, each of which your body needs, those in smaller amounts. Micronutrients are essential for the body's healthy daily operation.

The equation of calories in versus calories out is true; if you burn more calories than you eat, you will lose weight and vice versa. Some of you may be thinking, "Well, how does Lucy Lu eat so much more than me yet she's much leaner than me?" I'm glad you asked! Does Lucy Lu have a consistent exercise regimen? If she plays sports, is a regular at the ol' LA Fitness or something of the like, she's built a very efficient metabolism. Believe it or not, right at this moment you are burning calories, simply reading a book. I know, ground breaking news. Amazing, isn't it? As you may or may not know, muscle requires more units of energy per day to survive and function. The scientific definition of units of energy in this instance would be calories. Therefore, someone with more muscle would need or "be able to" eat more calories and stay at their current weight. Taking this one step further, as we mentioned in the exercise chapter, muscle takes the place of the fat, along with being denser than fat. Five pounds of muscle is visually smaller than five pounds of fat, causing someone with a higher percentage of muscle to appear "smaller," or "toned" as the kids like to call it these days. Calories are *great*, especially when you work *with* your body to keep it as efficient as possible.

The type and source of calories you eat truly does matter though. With this standard equation, you could technically lose weight eating only Reese's cups and potato chips, as long as your intake does not exceed your expenditure. However, this is obviously not healthy and keeps you from having the nutrition your body requires, puts you at risk of losing a high amount of muscle instead of fat, and can put you at risk for numerous illnesses, including diabetes. For this reason, I do not believe that going straight to a "counting" program or a predetermined meal program is beneficial. This could include counting points, calories, pre-cooked meals, and so on, using them without proper knowledge about why we're having those certain foods or how to stay truly healthy by abiding by these numbers. This is especially risky if you already have a dietary illness, such as diabetes. If one were to go to a "counting" program without proper knowledge of food to manage one's diabetes, they could potentially wreak havoc on their body, trying to manage it by eating too many carbohydrates of which a diabetic would need to be mindful of. They might be abiding by the counting program, but not abiding by their body's needs. This is why in my e-course "Thrive: Food, Fitness, and Life" not only do we delve into nutrition basics for *your* body type, but also understanding cravings and indulging in a healthy way for a life without deprivation, as well as why you might be reaching for foods to cope with stress, sadness, or other emotions. It's a package deal, not a matter of "yes" and "no" foods.

We need to have a basic understanding of what is in our food to find true health and feel our very best. Organic, non-GMO, and other stipulations such as these are important. A good rule of thumb for organic is "the dirty dozen." There are a dozen foods that should be eaten organically as often as possible to ensure you're not ingesting the chemicals and pesticides that can be harmful to your body. Same goes for non-GMO. If you can, opt for the non-GMO option. I don't think it's as important to go deep into these concepts here—I could literally write an entire other book on food quality, but we don't need to know that now. Be sure your food is of high-quality, grown naturally, from a trustworthy source, and your insides will thank you.

Macronutrients are especially helpful in creating your healthiest you, so let's talk about them. "Macro counting," as I mentioned I've done before, is a common phrase in the fitness industry at the moment. However, literally counting everything you put into your mouth is not at all necessary to have adequate amounts of each macronutrient for your health and body composition.

First, let's cover what each of the macronutrients does in the body. Protein composes most of the body. It is required for proper muscle building and repair. Outside of building muscle, protein is also necessary for:

- A healthy immune system
- Strong hair, skin, and nails
- Production of hormones

This is not an exhaustive list, but you can see how protein is necessary for proper bodily function, especially for fitness. It also plays a lead role in satiation.

Protein is made up of different amino acids, many of which the body can make on its own, and nine of which the body cannot. These nine are called "essential." Therefore, we must acquire essential amino acids through our food choices. Foods that contain all nine essential amino acids on their own are called complete proteins, and those that do not are called incomplete proteins. Complete protein examples include most animal sources such as:

- Eggs
- Poultry
- Beef
- Fish

There are plant-based sources as well, such as:

- Buckwheat
- Quinoa
- Chia seeds

Incomplete sources of protein can be combined with other incomplete sources to create a complete protein. For example, rice and beans together create a complete source of protein.

The most concentrated and easiest forms of protein do come from animal sources, but if you choose veganism or vegetarianism you can still obtain an adequate amount of protein—it may just take a bit more knowledge of what particular plant-based proteins you're consuming.

Lack of protein can cause brittle hair, poor skin, low energy, poor immune system functioning, and more.

There are guidelines as to how much protein a person needs, but these are highly individualized numbers. "The Dietary Reference Intake states that about 0.8 grams per kg of bodyweight" is suggested[13]. However, those who are more active require more protein, especially if they are trying to build muscle. A good rule of thumb is to include about a palm-size portion at each meal. That's it. Eat your protein, friends. Make it simple. Your body needs protein for muscle health and proper functioning, so be sure to include a source of protein in each meal and you are all set.

---

13 "Protein Intake – How Much Protein Should You Eat Per Day?" Health Line, (www.healthline.com/nutrition/how-much-protein-per-day).

Fat went through a phase when it was like the new kid at school that nobody liked so people stopped including it in their diets. It even went through a dreadful phase when food companies were actually removing the fat from their products to create "fat-free" food items by replacing the fat with sugar and chemicals. Not good, kids. Not good.

Fats are another main source of the body's energy; they are fundamental to proper brain functioning, supple hair and skin, the absorption of nutrients, as well as keeping you satiated throughout the day. They can be saturated, unsaturated, or trans fats. Trans fats are industrially-created and the only type that should be eliminated from the diet as much as possible as they are not natural sources and not efficiently used by the body. Trans fats are found in processed foods, fried foods, and many low-quality dessert items.

Let's keep it simple. Focus on high-quality sources of unsaturated fats, with some high-quality saturated fats a little less frequently.

High-quality sources of unsaturated fats:

- Olive oil

- Avocados

- Nuts and nut butters

- Seeds

High-quality sources of saturated fats:

- Beef

- Butter

- Coconut oil
- Full-fat dairy

Proper portioning of fats is said to be about the amount of two fingers in length, or 1-2 tablespoons. Because fat is more calorically dense, a serving size is smaller than that of a carbohydrate or protein. Furthermore, beef (and sometimes diary, like Greek yogurt) contain mostly protein in their macronutrient makeup, so the portion sizing is in line with that of a protein. Including a high-quality source of healthy fat into every meal is vital to be sure your body is receiving the proper amounts each day.

Carbohydrates seem to have a pretty bad reputation among the health-conscious these days. This isn't necessary, though. Carbohydrates are quite good for you when eating the proper source and quality. Carbohydrates are a plentiful source of fiber, which is necessary for regularity—ahem, your frequency in the bathroom—and regulating blood sugar, to name a few. Further, carbohydrates are one of the body's main sources of energy.

There are two types of carbohydrates:

- Simple
- Complex

Complex carbohydrates should make up the bulk of your carbohydrate consumption.

Complex indicates that they take the body longer to break down and provide a steady release of energy throughout the following few hours. Why does that matter? It keeps your energy high, without having that all-too-familiar afternoon crash a few hours later. Not only this but it regulates your blood sugar (hold tight, we're getting to why that's important).

Complex carbohydrates examples include:

- Whole grains
- Sweet potato and other starchy vegetables
- Leafy green vegetables

On the other hand, simple carbohydrates supply a quick burst of energy followed by a crash. A prime example of a simple carbohydrate is table sugar, however, fruits, sweeteners, and refined sugars found in processed foods and desserts are also simple carbohydrates. Although fruit is on this list, it also contains a wide variety of necessary micronutrients and should not be eliminated from your diet.

During the twentieth century, we began to heavily process many foods in order to increase their shelf life and lower the cost. We cheapened the food supply monetarily and nutritionally. During processing, food producers now will often take a complex carbohydrate and make it into a simple carbohydrate. For example, bread. A whole grain is made up of three different parts, two of which contain nutrients used by the body, and one that is just kind of there to keep things together. During the processing, the two parts containing nutrients are stripped, leaving only the third. The whole grain is now a simple carbohydrate. This is why processed foods are considered simple forms of carbohydrates. Many processed foods are actually quite far from being considered "food" at all. The true food has been eliminated and replaced with chemicals or sugar. These are commonly referred to as empty calories because your body cannot use them like it can a nutrient.

This is not to say that you should never ever eat processed foods. Life happens, balance is necessary. Try to eat mostly real, whole foods. If the bulk of your diet is made up of simple carbohydrates or processed foods, this could be they key reason you feel you need coffee through an IV in the afternoon or find yourself craving sugar on the regular. Subsisting on simple carbohydrates gives you only minimal bursts of energy, not sustained periods like complex carbohydrates do.

As you can see, the problem isn't carbohydrates themselves, but rather the source of carbohydrates you eat most frequently. Include about a fist-size of leafy vegetables and a fist-size of complex carbohydrates at each meal.

With this knowledge and these simple portion guidelines, creating balance with healthy eating and your lifestyle can be easy. When going out to a restaurant, simply fulfill the nutrients and it's simple as that! Furthermore, when eating out at restaurants, it is common to be served a serving size much larger than what it should be. Being aware of portion sizes helps finding balance much easier. Don't be afraid to ask for what you want. I prefer to order salads with the dressing on the side so I don't end up with four servings of dressing. You can also ask for your meat grilled or blackened instead of fried. You get to be in charge.

Now you can see why juice detoxes or eating only fruit and veggies can be harmful to your body. You're completely lacking many nutrients the body requires and causing it to go into starvation mode if you don't consume enough calories. You cannot outsmart your body. If you consume far too few calories, your body doesn't know you're trying to fit into that bikini for Hawaii and thinks you're in the middle of a desert, just you and your camel without a source of food anywhere nearby. So to make up for it, every time you do eat, it gets stored for later, your metabolism slows to not burn off your energy source, and it becomes even more difficult to lose fat. When it comes to juicing or things like a "water diet," (I actually saw an ad for that on Facebook today . . . no) just don't even think about doing them.

My greatest piece of advice is to learn to read the nutrition label, and not just for calories or macronutrient grams, but rather for the ingredients themselves. If the ingredients list is a mile long of things sounding like they were created in a lab, your body is probably just as confused when you eat them as your mind is when you try to pronounce them. Staying far away from packaged foods forever is a tall order, but with growing knowledge and awareness of this issue, more brands are creating packaged foods that are full of whole and nutritious ingredients. Most of the time, be sure that your ingredients list contains mostly real foods from the earth.

Secondly, read the nutrition labels for portion sizes. Most Americans consume far more than what a true serving size should be. By understanding servings sizes, it's easier to feel in charge of what you're eating when you're at restaurants or friends' houses. For example, a serving size of salad dressing is generally two tablespoons. However, a salad is rarely served with just two tablespoons. But remember, you get to be in charge. If you're tired of vinaigrette and just want the damn ranch already, order it on the side. Opt to dip each bite or pour some on yourself so you know you're not eating hundreds of empty calories in dressing alone.

See? So far, so good. We're keeping it nice and simple! It doesn't have to be hard! I'm about to get a tad scientific, but just to show you why you might be craving Ben and Jerry's every day, falling asleep at your desk, or feeling constantly hungry. We're talking blood sugar levels. The sneaky little guys that make you go from bouncing off the walls to needing a nap in no time flat.

When we eat, carbohydrates are broken down into glucose, causing blood sugar to rise. This presence of glucose in the bloodstream signals the release of insulin, the hormone responsible for bringing blood sugar back to normal by allowing the glucose to be used for energy. Any excess glucose not used for energy is stored for later. The presence of protein, fiber, and healthy fat also slow the release of glucose to provide a steadier source of energy to the body and regulate blood sugar.

The issue is how the processing of our foods has become so mainstream that most people are used to eating high amounts of simple carbohydrates (quick release of sugar into the blood) and our bodies have become *too good* at releasing insulin. Often, too much insulin is released and our blood sugar levels are brought down too low. This signals to your brain that you need energy! The quickest form of energy? You guessed it, sugar. This is a very simple explanation as to why you may constantly be craving sweets and lower quality carbohydrates—your blood sugar is simply out of whack. Try adding more fibrous veggies and less processed foods into your diet and watch your cravings subside.

This also explains feeling exceptionally tired in the

afternoon after a big lunch or having to go for that third cup of coffee in the early afternoon. Your body is so busy trying to break down and digest your food that there's no energy left to look at your fifty-seventh spreadsheet Bob needs you to take care of.

When you create each meal to include a portion of protein, healthy fat, and complex carbohydrate (if not with veggies, be sure to include a veggie as well—don't forget those mircos!) your body can more easily process the meal to provide a steady release of energy throughout the day, as opposed to a quick burst of energy followed by a crash from a meal lacking balanced macro nutrition. By adding more balance into your meals you will begin to have more energy, sleep more deeply, feel fuller longer, experience healthier cravings, and shed excess weight your body no longer needs. Look to the end of this chapter for an example of a balanced plate.

Healthier cravings, did that grab your attention? I thought it might. It's just the same as when you go out for a weekend of fun food and dessert every day, you come home and you find your cravings for junk food off the wall—like a puppy that just found an empty jar of peanut butter. I nailed it, didn't I? The more low-quality foods you eat, the more you crave them. Same goes for healthier foods. When you eat more high-quality foods, full of colorful fruits and vegetables, your brain gets a "light bulb moment." When you fuel your body in a way that it can use all of the food for energy and everything operates smoothly, you feel great. You're more alert—no foggy brain, you sleep better, have a more positive mood, and so much more. Your brain says, "Wait a minute, this is how it's supposed to work! Give me more of that," and you find yourself craving healthier foods more and more. This is why for those who have gotten into a healthy lifestyle, when they have a few less than nutritious foods their brain says, "Alright that was delicious but I really need some vegetables now," and you crave healthier foods after weekends like this. Jackpot! Healthy made easy!

To get you to that point, I have a little secret to "resetting" your body after one of those necessary life moments like a night on the town or a weekend in Napa Valley. Okay, okay. It's not really a secret. This could be referred to as resetting your body to its factory settings. Meaning, get your insides back to the point where they were created to operate. This way, you feel your best physically *and* mentally, and your waistline may thank you as well.

As you already know, the body needs a combination of each of the three macronutrients. Furthermore, each time you eat, your blood sugar rises (varying degrees depending on numerous factors such as what types and how much) and your body does what it knows how to do to bring it back down to normal. Often times, eating less than nutritious things might include one or a combination of heavy carbs, heavy processed foods, alcohol, sweet treats, and so on. After a meal such as this, your blood sugar spikes much more than normal and it sends you on a drastic blood sugar roller coaster. To balance this out, and here's the trick, a simple adjustment to your next meal (or few) is helpful: Reduce your carbohydrate intake and increase your fibrous veggies (i.e., leafy greens, if possible) at the next meal. Skip the side of fruit with your veggie omelet or add some avocado to your omelet instead of the English muffin. This will reduce your intake of carbohydrate and subsequent glucose into the blood, naturally bringing your blood sugar levels back to normal. When I work with clients and we gain an understanding of *their own* body, it becomes much easier to know what these portion adjustments might look like, as well as other simple changes that can regulate blood sugar as well in their daily routine.

The blood sugar roller coaster might be why people often set out for a diet style such as vegan, and still feel as though they're either gaining weight, lacking energy, or both. This is because eating vegan doesn't automatically make each food item high-quality or low-sugar. It can still contain a high amount of refined sugar, sending you on the blood sugar roller coaster. For example, Oreos are vegan. Going vegan improperly, by eating too many of the less-than-nutritious-yet-vegan foods, could cause you to not receive adequate amounts of fiber, fat, or other nutrient deficiencies. Veganism is not bad, and if that's what you choose, great. Just be sure to educate yourself on proper, nutritious, vegan-friendly foods to fulfill all macronutrient needs. This goes for any "style" of eating. I believe in no foods being off-limits, so I'm not an advocate for any "style" in particular if it makes you feel fantastic. Many individuals choose one for ethical or other reasons, but just keep this in mind.

Sleep is a non-negotiable for helping your body reach peak performance along with your nutrition. When we do not get an adequate amount of sleep, our bodies search for any source of energy they can find. Most people either end up drinking their body weight in coffee or energy drinks or eating more. Your brain sends a signal to your mind that it needs energy. So, without adequate sleep, your brain may begin to ask your body for energy in the form of food instead.

By cleaning up your diet, not only are you adding years to your life by preventing disease and illness, but you're also fueling your mind to help you achieve the best life you possibly can. By eating nutritiously, you're managing sleep, cravings, stress, and peace of mind.

It can be simple. You don't have to track every single thing you put into your mouth to be successful. Begin by making correlations between the foods you eat and the way you feel each day and learn to truly listen *and respond* to what your body needs and wants. The action steps will help you do this. This makes it sound like you're beginning a new romantic relationship with someone you're infatuated with, and I guess that's what it should feel like. Decide to care for yourself so much that you do everything you can to keep it loved, healthy, and happy.

I totally understand that there is so much conflicting information out there, making it easy to become discouraged and unsure of what to do. I felt the exact same way for years. As a matter of fact, two of my favorite leaders in the nutrition and wellness industry today have conflicting views and research to support both of them. When I decided I needed to make a shift and focus on all-encompassing *health,* I looked to simplicity first. What I've included here for you is all you need to find nutritional balance, know you're fueling your body exquisitely, and finally conclude the internal battle of which rules to follow next. Everything explained above is simply science, and when you learn to work with the science of your body, you truly cannot mess up. Create a balance of what you know and what feels best physically *and* mentally.

High-quality food is imperative, but so is high-quality

peace of mind. Don't expect yourself to never have another french fry, or only allow yourself to have them on Saturdays. That is *not* healthy nor is it balance. Allowing less than nutritious foods only on the weekends is simply another rule. Get rid of the rigid rules. Balance is eating nutritious, high-quality foods *most* of the time. For some of you, that may mean the popular 80/20 rule—eating high-quality 80 percent of the time and less than nutritious 20 percent of the time. For some of you that may mean 90/10 or 70/30. Experiment to discover what makes you feel free, strong, healthy, happy, and like the best version of yourself that you can be. Go through your days eating meals you love, things you crave (nutritious or non, but mostly nutritious), and make the effort to be the healthiest version of yourself inside *and* out.

At first, this may feel daunting and a bit scary. You may not trust yourself to be able to follow through. If that is the case, *decide* to believe in yourself. Give yourself permission to try. Create a vivid vision of the highest version of yourself and begin to act like her every single day. Truly *believe* you can do it. I will, however, *always* recommend hiring a coach for guidance at first to keep your mindset healthy and in the proper direction, as well as to learn how to discover what truly does work best for you, your body, and your mind. Here are the action steps to master nutrition for a healthy body *and* mind:

1. Commit yourself to being truly healthy.

Choose high-quality foods because you know it's what's best for your body, while also having an ice cream cone or cocktail every now and then if that's what you love. Life is meant to be enjoyed. Refrain from creating strict rules when it comes to food. *This* is true health. When you create a healthy nutrition and exercise plan coupled with a strong and positive mindset, oh, my dear, that is ultimate health.

2. Ingredient swaps

It can be difficult to stop craving all things burgers, burritos, and cupcakes. When you're wanting to be a little more nutritious, but that-less-than-nutritious food just sounds so good, my secret weapon is ingredient swaps. With the growing interest in nutrition and health, there are so many recipe developers who create your average less-than-nutritious meals a little healthier. From french fries and chicken fingers to donuts and cheesecake, there are a myriad of resources to help you swap the often highly-processed ingredients with more high-quality, better-for-you ingredients. Satisfy your craving without wreaking havoc on your insides. The e-course "Thrive: Food, Fitness, and Life" offers participants numerous tools to make this not only successful, but tasty and enjoyable with things like an ingredient swap list and numerous "healthified" recipes.

3. Discover why you want to do this and start working towards *that.*

So, you want to eat healthier. You want to clean up your diet, possibly shed excess weight, or gain some healthy pounds.

Why? Why do you want to be healthier? What will it bring into your life that you don't feel you have right now? How will that change your life? Mentally, spiritually, financially, in relationships, in your career—how will achieving that change every single area of your life?

Now work towards *that*. Not a number on the scale or size of your jeans. Work for the person *in* the jeans. If the highest version of yourself does not manage stress with an afternoon brownie, how does she? If the highest version of you takes a stressful day and puts a smile on anyway because she's grateful for everything she *does* have, focusing on the positive instead of the negative, then start acting like her. If the highest version of you decides to make a homemade taco instead of hitting the drive-through at Taco Bell, do it. She might also include a little dessert every now and then or let loose at brunch on Sunday at her favorite spot. The highest version of yourself probably does fuel herself wonderfully, but what else does she do?

This is the key to truly creating a lifestyle shift. This is your motivation for choosing the veggie-packed delicious dinner over the small cheeseburger that might fit your calories. Commit to thriving, inside and out.

These simple mindset shifts are a crucial component in your overall success. When you consistently focus on what you're doing well and keep your mood high and optimistic, choosing healthier options becomes more natural. It becomes *just what you do*. Because let's face it, by picking up this book you've already decided to be the very best version of yourself, so you already are her. Make decisions as her.

4. Pick your battles.

A critical decision that made finding my version of balance so much easier was picking my battles with nutrition. If you literally cut out every single thing that is said to have some sort of a negative impact related to it, there wouldn't be much left to eat and that would feel incredibly restrictive. So I pick my battles. I choose to abide by the dirty-dozen and clean-fifteen organic guidelines, as well as investing in organic meat. Sometimes I choose a sugar-free vanilla latte (also known as the chemical infested one) instead of the real deal. And yes, I do understand that those chemicals are horrible for me, but remember, it's not a daily occurrence. I have the occasional diet coke (ugh, that fizz on a hot day). I choose dairy-free instead of dairy because it just isn't worth the pain I experience when I have dairy. Sometimes I choose fries for a side instead of veggies. Most of the time I choose real whole foods, but I also want to live my life. If I want a darn side of fries by golly I'm going to get them. In a perfect world, all of my food would be top-notch quality, and I'd only ever choose the whole foods that are best for me. But imperfection is okay. Imperfection makes you human. Balance is choosing when to be imperfect. It's choosing what's important to you and learning what exactly your less-than-nutritious 20 percent consists of. Balance helps you sustain your healthiest lifestyle, inside and out. Decide what's important to you, decide what makes you feel best, and trust yourself that you've made the right decision.

Some might argue that eating high-quality most of the time is too expensive, so pick your battles. Instead of running through the drive through or picking up takeout, purchasing your own ingredients to make it will always be cheaper. Can't get meat *and* produce organic? Choose one. Purchase frozen organic fruits or veggies as they're almost always much cheaper. Purchase locally and in-season to bring the cost down. There is always a way. It's up to *you* to believe there *is* a way and choose what works for you.

5. Make nutritional correlations.

Earlier I mentioned that tracking my food was unhealthy for me. I did not set myself up with the proper mindset or outlook as to *why* I was tracking my food. Back then, it was purely for the number on the scale and the number of muscles I could see. I made zero correlation between how different macros or food sources made my body *feel*.

Instead, be mindful about how certain food sources affect your day to day. Do they deplete your energy or add to it? Do you sleep better or worse? Do you stay full or no? Make correlations to your energy levels, fullness, and mood. This can help you to keep away from certain foods because they don't make you feel your best. Earlier I mentioned I don't eat dairy and I'm mostly refined sugar-free. I'm lactose intolerant and don't feel well most of the time after eating a sugar-filled dessert. That doesn't mean I *never* have dessert, it just means I'm more intentional when I do.

There is quite the craze right now for cutting out certain food groups. On the one hand, I totally believe in it for a predetermined period of time, for the intention of understanding your own body and discovering what may or may not keep you feeling your best. Or possibly on occasion for a week or so to naturally "reset" your body if you're feeling less than your best. After all, that's how I figured out my food sensitivity issues. But just because Susie the Instagram model doesn't eat gluten doesn't mean that you have to cut out gluten to build a body you're confident in. If gluten makes you break out, or causes you to get overly tired then yes, by all means, reduce or cut it out. We are all different, so eating a certain way purely because so and so does and you would like a body like hers does not mean it will work that way *for you*. As a matter of fact, there are many different ways to discover what does work best in your body. In the e-course "Thrive: Food, Fitness, and Life," I show you how to do this in a balanced, simple, and healthy way. Head to www.dianamatuszak.com/work-with-me/ to download the e-course.

Furthermore, understanding the difference between high and low quality is imperative—meaning, the one with ingredients only from the earth instead of the one with added sugars and preservatives. Learn to understand what makes you feel your best, and that is all you need to do.

This could mean creating a journal to keep track or possibly purchasing one, however, if you find yourself a bit more naturally rigid or strict, or if you find yourself constantly making lists and your mood is easily affected when the list doesn't go as planned, I suggest *not* literally writing things down. Some people (me included) have a more obsessive or addictive personality and we find happiness in doing things perfectly. Tracking everything may begin to cause more harm than good. Instead, make an effort to be more mindful. Pay more attention to yourself around meal time and throughout the day. Notice what you ate on days you felt great. Notice what you ate (or didn't eat) on days you felt depleted. Doing this will help make the necessary correlations.

6. Your hunger and fullness cues

When we become disconnected from our biological hunger and fullness cues, it can be easy to overeat, or simply eat by the clock. Many fitness regimens suggest eating a certain amount a certain amount of time after or before a workout, or every three hours, and so on. Instead, I encourage you to become very in tune with your own hunger and fullness cues. Ask yourself these questions:

Am I eating because I'm hungry? Or because it's noon?

Am I eating because I'm hungry or because it's in front of me?

Am I not eating because it's not dinner time yet even though I'm starving? Causing me to overeat come dinner and feel uncomfortably full later?

These simple questions can help you learn to know your body's signals and respond to them appropriately. Generally, eat when you're hungry and stop when you're satisfied and comfortably full. Remember, this is not an overnight skill. You may have years of not truly listening to your body; don't beat yourself up if this seems really difficult. Soon, you will understand and be able to follow through.

7. Hire a coach.

In this chapter, I simplified it for you. But often times, it is beneficial for people to hire a coach when beginning these new habits, especially while discovering which foods work best in your body. For example, some people operate really well a higher carbohydrate diet, while others operate well on a higher fatty protein diet. Having guidance and support to understand your body's signals and correlations speeds up this process. Not to mention a mentor or helping-hand in keeping your mindset positive and self-serving, as well as factoring in your life's other unique demands speeds up the process of creating the very best version of you.

If you'd like, head to my website (www.dianamatuszak. com) to schedule a food and fitness assessment and get aligned with your unique pathway.

Food is another area where my point of view differs from others in my field. Yes, you 100 percent need to love yourself in every way to be successful, no matter what stage you're in. But if you're constantly uncomfortable in your own skin, get easily winded when you exercise, have horrible energy or sleep . . . then you *need* to look at the way you eat. This specifically is where my point of view differs from others in my field—I do think changing food habits to achieve your most confident body is healthy, *when coming from healthy intentions.* If you have goals to be the most confident version of yourself out of love for *you* and a desire to be the best version of yourself that you were created to be, then that's great. But doing so in a manner where no foods are off limits, keeping your happiness a number one priority, and staying focused on your *true* goals (more confidence, to be alive and healthy into old age, to have more energy to go after life goals . . .) not what your body *looks* like.

That is who I am, and who I try to be every day. I don't eat dairy because it makes me feel like a pregnant whale which doesn't help me be my best self, but I wouldn't have known this if I didn't experiment with it. Just like growing a booty like JLo requires strengthening your booty muscles, so does strengthening your willpower and motivation to discover your healthiest balance until it's a habit for you.

It might be easy to feel overwhelmed by nutrition. My hope is that this chapter showed you how to create your version of a healthy balance, cleared up your confusion, and helped you see through the fog. It can be simple, but it's up to you to make it so. Include a serving of high-quality protein, fat, fibrous carbohydrate, and vegetable in each meal—that's it. See, it really is possible to hate kale and still be healthy! Establish these balanced healthy habits as if you are already the best version of you, until they're simply what you do. You'll be well on your way to living your best life.

BALANCED PLATE

Keys To Success:

- *Flexibility not Rigidity:* Different macronutrient needs are unique to each individual. Allow this template to shift and change as you learn more about what foods and food combinations make you feel your best!
- *Portions:* Refer to portion suggestions using the your hand.
- *Eat Until Satisfied:* listen to your body's signals. Eat until you feel energized. not too little and not too much. About 80% full.

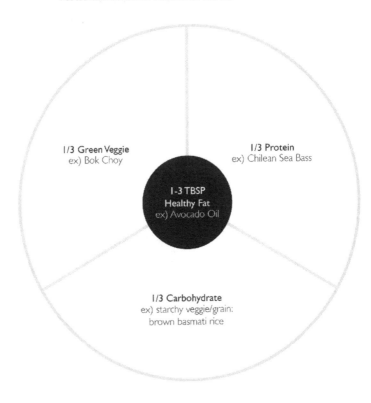

1/3 Green Veggie
ex) Bok Choy

1/3 Protein
ex) Chilean Sea Bass

1-3 TBSP
Healthy Fat
ex) Avocado Oil

1/3 Carbohydrate
ex) starchy veggie/grain:
brown basmati rice

CHAPTER 7

Spending tonight with my two favorite men, Ben and Jerry.

"Living a healthier lifestyle is about more than losing weight, it's about losing the mindset that got you there in the first place."

—Elle Sommer

WHAT DO ALL romantic comedies have in common? You know what I mean—the ones where there is a breakup between two love-birds who weren't really meant to be together before the good part of the movie when she meets her new soulmate and it's all roses and cutesy butterfly feelings?

You guessed it: ice cream, wine, or a combination of the two. It's ingrained in our brains that a woman's breakup is immediately followed by a sleepover with her friends where they get drunk on wine or dig into a pint of Ben and Jerry's while talking about what a jerk he was anyway.

On the other hand, it might look like friends *trying* to get her to go out to eat with them or go to happy hour to get her spirits back, but she's too sad to eat anything, even banana foster pancakes with homemade caramel frosting at her favorite brunch spot.

Most of us learn this coping method of manipulating food early in our childhood as away of dealing with all things sad, emotional, or stressful. Whether it's from being given a snack to make you stop crying as a toddler (regardless of whether you were hungry), watching one of those rom-coms, observing your mom eat noticeably less out of nerves for her work presentation, or something else along the way. The positive intention of helping yourself feel better is there, but this solution is ready for an up-level.

For some, their crutch is eating more. For others, it's not eating at all. Let's dig into why so many of us turn to Ben and Jerry or Mr. Orville Redenbacher after a stressful week at work, or why some of us can't even look at them at all.

Right now, I'm going to have to ask you to get a piece of paper and a pen and get ready to write. This is a not-so-obvious step we need to cover before digging into why so many of us turn to Ben and Jerry to fix our problems. We're going to create a vision of your best life so clear you can taste the California-fresh almond butter over your perfect California-fresh green smoothie bowl. Let your heart guide you, ignite what truly makes you happy, and with collaboration from God or your source, let your highest self come to life.

Answer the following questions from the highest version of yourself:

1. If you had your absolute dream career, what would it be? Not what Mom wants you to do, not what you think you should do—what do you truly want to do?

2. If you could go anywhere or live anywhere, where would it be?

3. If money were no object, what would you study, where would you travel, what amazing things would you allow yourself to do?

4. If you were living as the highest version of yourself, how would you act? Happier? More lighthearted? More compassionate? Bolder? More confident?

5. What would you believe about yourself? About your capabilities, your drive?

6. What would you be proud of?

7. How would you go about every day? How would you go about daily tasks like laundry or dishes?

8. What would your values be?

9. How would you respond to difficult situations?

10. What else does the highest version of you think, believe, do?

Write anything else that comes to mind, painting a vivid picture of the very best version of you. Note how she thinks, what she believes, and who she hangs out with. How she nourishes her body. Anything that helps paint the picture of your best life, as the best version of you just a pinch clearer.

Take a moment to picture yourself going through an ideal day as this person. Notice how it feels, even just for a moment, to live as that version of you. Do you see the gaps between the you that's here today and the highest version of yourself? This is a judgment-free exercise. Just simply be curious and notice. If judgments come up, say, "Thanks, meanie, but I don't need you right now. You come up too often as it is." Simply allow yourself to be inquisitive.

I'm guessing now you can clearly see the gap between the person you are today and the person you are trying to be, rather than the person you were born to be. You are the only *you* that will ever be born. Why not be the very best version of you? You may or may not see clear action steps to get you from where you are to where you want to be. If you do, that is fantastic! If not, you're in the right place! Either way, after a few changes (some big, some small), you will be empowered to live as that best version of you!

I want you to continue to goal-set and dream and do what you can to become that version of yourself. But there are some problems that come along with it, which you might even be experiencing right now, holding you back from truly living as her. Don't worry, I went through these too and I'm going to show you how to course-correct or completely avoid them. This is where we dig in. I'm going to show you an approach to "manipulating" food you probably don't quite see coming, but I believe it's a major player in the development of self-disappointment, dissatisfaction, and stress that we tend to overlook when dealing with emotional eating (or not eating).

The problem is that many of us get so excited about being this new version of ourselves, almost *too* excited. We can see her clearly, we can almost feel it. We might identify the things we need to change in order to be her. If you're like me, the issue is that we go balls to the wall for these things. We go all in. At first glance, this doesn't appear to be a negative thing. Sometimes it's not, but often times it is. We try to change every little thing we don't like, everything that isn't matching the highest version of ourselves, and we try to be sure to leave nothing behind. We wake up on Monday and change every little thing, swearing to never be our old selves again.

And then? We crash. We can't sustain the massive 180 we just took, and we revert back to our old ways, often with massive feelings of despair, disappointment, and even disgust with ourselves. I've been there, done that, got the shirt. Many times.

Instead of going all in, maybe you look at those things and go, "Yeah right, that's a whole lot of change and sounds way too overwhelming right now." So you say maybe next year, or when you have enough money, or when you have abs, or when you have a tall, dark, and handsome husband, or whenever x happens, justifying why you can't do it until _____. You go into freeze mode and don't even start at all.

Whichever side you find yourself on, let's examine how that might correlate with your food habits that are holding you back from being the highest version of you mind, body, and soul.

I used to wake up on Monday for what seemed like the hundredth time, swearing that this time, beginning today (again), it would be different. The binge eating would stop. I would finally be free from food. After years of restriction having turned into binging, I'd finally had it. I'd look to do everything in my power to make it stop.

The day would seem to go well—I'd have a healthy breakfast I loved, then a nourishing lunch and dinner, but then evening would come. There would be an entirely new person inside of me and the binging would come back as fast as you can say, "Where's the pantry?" I didn't feel I had control over my own thoughts or impulses anymore. I was completely consumed with thoughts of food, unable to make them go away until the feelings of disgust and guilt would overwhelm me in their place. I'd created a monster. And what was worse, before my freshman year weight-gain, I'd never before understood that I previously experienced issues with food. What I didn't realize was that my younger self—counting the number of foods eaten that day on her hand—had no idea that she had an issue with food. I would think, "There's no way I could have an issue with food, I love eating too much." But then I created fierce rules around what I could and couldn't eat, causing me to restrict heavily. This eventually led me to over-eating because I was so focused on under-eating or "dieting." Then I understood those who struggled around food. I'd not only experienced one side, but the opposite as well. For me, it truly is as if there is an entirely different person in my mind taking over all thoughts and decisions.

At the end of freshman year when I decided I wanted to grab ahold of my nutrition and body, I didn't quite understand how my 180 degree Monday-morning efforts could be a bad thing. Moreover, I didn't quite see that I was even trying to make a 180. I thought I was being a go-getter, not taking failure as an option. It's the way I'd always been. Captain of my sports teams, valedictorian of my high school, academic awards and scholarships in college—going all-in is written into my blood. What I didn't realize was I'd gone too far trying to completely transform myself to achieve the happiness I wanted, the relationships I wanted, and to be the person I so badly wanted to be, thinking other people might like me better (key detail). I believed that having the "dream body" was the best way to get there. It took me quite some time to realize how strongly I'd been neglecting my cravings and even the nutritious foods I loved because I *needed* to abide by every single rule. I wanted that body, I wanted that life, and I wanted it right away, regardless of the toll it would take on my wellbeing and happiness on the way there.

When it finally came time to let myself choose balance after *deciding* I didn't have to be that strict—that it was possible to find balance *and* pride in my own body—all hell had already broken loose. It began with just a couple of binges. But soon, it was a daily occurrence. I could not be trusted around anything that was previously on my list of "no's" when it came to foods I'd allow myself to eat. The monster inside of me was sort of like the cookie monster but she liked literally everything in large quantities and wasn't very nice. I joke about it now. But then? It caused me pain like I'd never experienced before, pain I wouldn't wish upon my worst enemy. It pushed me into the worst mental space I'd ever been in my life, hardly able to pull myself out of it. I finally understood the mental and emotional struggles I previously couldn't grasp.

One serving of chips turned into my hand in the bag

until it was gone, telling myself that once the bag was gone, I just wouldn't buy them again. The following day, I would find myself buying the chips again, saying I'd learn to only have one serving instead. A spoonful of peanut butter turned into a spoon in the jar. And the cycle repeated itself, spiraling further and further down until I could hardly see a way out. I continued to be harder on myself. My friends didn't understand what I was going through. I kept them away from me, and I felt lonelier than ever. I was unhappy in numerous areas of my life, using food to cope. There were so many things I wanted so badly—a really strong relationship with my friends and a sense of true connection where people loved me for *me*. I didn't really enjoy getting drunk or staying out late partying as college continued on, and I felt like an outcast. I didn't think people liked me as much because I didn't enjoy those things like most people did, but ignoring it and covering it up in unhealthy ways made it all easier for me. Feeling stressed, overwhelmed, sad—it all made me want to eat more. One problem was fueling another.

Some of you may have a very similar experience to me. You may have experienced accidental (or purposeful) restriction leading to binging that became much worse. Or maybe you resonate with me on feelings of disappointment, stress, or sadness leading you to the pantry as if it's going to give you a hug. On the other hand, maybe your response to these things is to not eat, as if that's the only thing you feel you do have control over. Either way, it's using food to numb-out or stop feeling what your body is telling you needs attention. Giving attention to what it needs can feel too hard. For instance, "Should I think about my horrible relationship and actually confront it? Or schedule a meeting with my boss who's treating me like a pile of horse doo doo? Food is much easier . . ."

Often we expect too much from ourselves. We get really excited about growing and evolving into a better version of ourselves, identify the necessary changes, that we try to change them all at once. Or we get scared and run away completely, heading back to the food for healing instead. Helga is not a fan of change and she lends a helping hand in fueling our bad habits. Being motivated is a very good thing, but our efforts to find success must be *balanced*. Excitement and motivation are fabulous, but let's savor them over the course of every day instead of turning from potato chip couch junkie into broccoli-loving triathlon runner. When we just can't sustain our skyscraper-level of a bar we have set for ourselves, we become angry and criticize ourselves for not being able to follow through.

Instead of it looking like a nearly impossible task, let's first break it down. Allow yourself and your life to be balanced, and tackle one thing at a time. This goes for efforts towards creating a new healthy lifestyle, forming a new habit, or breaking an old one. This can be applied to all areas of life, not just food and exercise. Recall back to the dream life we just envisioned above. Allow that vision to be your guide in breaking it all down and deciding what step to take first.

If you're on the go-getter side, the answer is not to just keep trudging along, trying to continue to "just stop" doing the things you want to stop doing so often, or if you're on the other side, just running from it and trying to will your disappointment away is not the answer either. So what *is* the answer? The answer is to address the root of the issue itself that we are trying so hard to improve and be willing to take the steps to improve *that*.

Many of my clients have experienced emotional eating. The one thing they all have in common is stress stemming from multiple areas of their lives. They might cope with the stress by numbing out with food, completely frustrated and outraged they are unable to "just stop eating," or they might cope with stress by skipping meals in an effort to control something when their life feels out of control.

When people who haven't ever experienced major issues with food say, "Well, if they'd just stop eating they'd lose weight," I get so angry my face turns the color of a tomato and I have smoke coming out of my ears like a real-life cartoon character. On one hand, some people do literally stop eating, as I've been mentioning. That is not at all healthy, not even a smidgen, nor is it the answer. It brings along with it a myriad of other problems. Secondly, would you tell a chain-smoker to "just stop smoking?" Would you tell an alcoholic to "just stop drinking?" No. Of course not. Using food as a coping tool is just as hardwired and addictive as these habits for many people. For them, food is a dependency and substance abuse just as the others are.

According to food addiction institute, "Food addiction is just like drug and alcohol addiction. Addiction means the body has become chemically dependent on one or more substances and needs these substances to function 'normally.' So when we are talking about a specific food as potentially being a substance of abuse, we are saying that the body has become dependent on a particular food or eating behavior. The most common addictive foods are foods high in sugar, flour, fat, grains and salt or some combination of these[14]."

When we eat many of these "trigger foods," the brain releases dopamine, which is what causes feelings of comfort or happiness, much like being with a loved one does. This motivates us to do this again and again because our brain tells us "this makes me feel better." Over time, it takes more food to create the same reaction, causing these episodes to become more and more intense. Thus far, following a difficult or stressful situation, eating to release dopamine is the best solution to this problem we've found, and as you can see, it becomes addictive. If individuals with a dependency on food could "just stop eating" during these situations, they would. It's not their fault, it's a change in their brains. So let's stop saying that.

Emotional eating often prevents us from making the lasting changes we truly want. If professional help isn't quite needed (see end of chapter for clarification), but you're constantly feeling discouraged and self-critical, how do you make this endless cycle stop? You travel to India, find the huge statue of Buddha and ask him to make it go away. I'm totally kidding, but a trip to India could be fun.

The truth is, often when we're dissatisfied with any area of our lives, we try to make up for the lost happiness in other ways. Helga reminds us that food (or lack thereof) can be a source of relief or joy from a very young age, which we bring into adulthood. Overwhelming stress at work turns

---

14 "What is Food Addiction," Food Addiction Institute, (https://foodaddictioninstitute.org/what-is-food-addiction/).

into daily evening numbing out with food, or an afternoon trip to the donuts in the break room. These acts aren't out of hunger, they're out of a search for relief.

In reality, we may be:

- Taking on too much at work and need to ask for an adjustment, or possibly hire help (at work or at home).

- Our marriage or relationship is not going well, causing feelings of stress, sadness, or loneliness.

- We're dissatisfied with our career path, lacking fulfillment or challenge.

- We don't have quality friendships or romantic relationships to spend time with and add to our quality of life.

- We're exhausted from poor lifestyle habits.

- We feel overwhelmed and lack a connection to God, or that which is greater.

- We "don't have time" for creativity that brings us true joy.

When we find the root of the issue and identify the triggers or situations that cause us to want to choose an unhealthy outlet, we find the thing that truly needs attention. When we are able to give much-needed attention to what is truly hurting, our dependency on food can release.

As I've mentioned, just as using food to numb out is our body's best answer to coping with difficulty, so is not eating. For example:

- "Well, if I just had a thinner body, he'd love me more," for relationship issues.

- "Well, if I just don't eat lunch—I'm too stressed to eat anyway—then I'll have this project done and I'll have more recognition at work," for career dissatisfaction.

- "Well, I don't have much control over many things right now, everything is falling apart, but I do have control over how much I eat (or don't)" for many dissatisfactions.

Food is often the first answer we find, but food is never the *true* answer to happiness.

I've had many clients who experience the emotional overeating end of the spectrum. After years and years of using food to numb out and cover up dissatisfaction, it can be astonishing to realize that that is actually *not* focusing on the food itself to lose the emotional eating weight. Searching for the next fad diet is far from the answer, so three cheers for not having to go through that again! This goes for whichever side of the spectrum you're on. So often when we struggle with emotional eating, we think dieting is the answer. "Well, if I could just stop eating sweets." When sweets are your answer to stress, it's really not about the sweets. Instead, we must shift our attention to the thing that is *causing* the stress that beckons the sweets response. Look to the action steps at the end of this chapter to hop on the train to no longer avoiding the problem (in the least scary way possible) and head straight to the town of living your best life you imagined above.

The only diet you ever need to go on is the one where you eat the foods you love—mostly nutritious and from the earth— balancing your meals and fueling your best days. Insider tip: when you do this, you feel so great you actually start to overflow happiness into the areas of life you're dissatisfied with. This sounds like the land of rainbows and unicorns, but I assure you it's not. Or maybe it is, and it just so happens that not so many people allow themselves to live there. But you do. You deserve that.

Some of you may be saying, "Well, I understand that, but I don't think I emotionally eat or restrict like that." By golly my dolly, I hope you don't. The truth is, you're reading this book, so there is a part of you that feels you're not quite being the best version of yourself yet. For those of you feeling this way, do you often set high expectations for yourself to become a better version of yourself and either end up giving up because it's too much, or not even start because it's too overwhelming? This is especially common with fitness and body image. If so, the answer is still found here by discovering the things that identify the difference between the version of yourself here now, and the version of yourself that you truly want to be—the highest version of you.

For example, a client of mine named Emma said during one of our sessions, "I didn't realize how much emotional attachment I had to certain foods. I've realized your stomach is controlled by your brain, and your brain can cope with mental challenges." Once we give our mind the permission to do the coping, then we truly make changes.

This week, add to your journaling any situations (stress, sadness, happiness) that cause you to crave or go for certain foods or unhealthy behaviors. Create a sense of hyper self-awareness and follow the steps below.

After years of restriction, food became my emotional crutch through binging. After pursuing multiple forms of self-growth and development, I began to grab ahold of my horrible relationship with food and my body. I discovered that I had thought finding the "dream body" would bring me all of the things I truly wanted. I wanted a relationship with someone that desired me. I wanted people to love the real me. I wanted to be myself and feel confident doing so. I wanted to find true happiness in every day and stop being my own worst critic. I wanted to be the best version of me in every way.

So how do you stop covering up these types of issues? How do you stop convincing yourself you can't be the highest version of you, and covering it up with food or lack thereof?

1. Forgive yourself.

Throw the F bomb around like confetti, again. Like a three-year-old's birthday party with a piñata raining confetti and sparkles, this book has you throwing that word around like your life depends on it. But actually, it does. Remaining angry at yourself for not being able to follow through or stop using these unhealthy habits is not helping you to change them. Instead, understand that this response is simply the best option that you have found thus far, stemming from learned habits as a young child that darn Helga has reinforced your entire life. But now, you're ready to up-level. You're ready and equipped with the knowledge, support, and belief in yourself that now is your time to flourish.

The impact of writing things down is so underrated, so I hope this book has helped you to find the power in it. Right now, write down this sentence: "I am powerful, I am capable, I am worthy, I deserve happiness in all areas of life, I am confident, I am the very best version of me." Next to that, write down, "I commit to _____" and write what you commit to doing from this day forward to help yourself address the things in your life that aren't at their best. However, do not write "I will not xxx." Instead write what you *will* do. This keeps your eye on the prize, honey, elevating your mood and keeping optimism at a prime!

2. Identify what truly needs improvement.

These might be considered your "triggers." What are the situations, seasons, people, habits, or anything else that cause your eat-to-numb/don't-eat-to-numb response to turn on? Begin with the smallest, least intimidating one and move onto the bigger ones. Focus on one at a time. Identify the easiest one to conquer first. When this trigger or situation comes up, what are you going to do instead, or how are you going to prevent it? What needs to be in place to ensure that you follow through with your healthier habit instead? Once you have conquered that one, move onto the next one, slowly working one by one until you reach the biggest. My e-course "Thrive: Food, Fitness, and Life" offers guidance and simple to implement mechanisms to help discover what needs improvement, and how to manage it during the phase of putting in work to improve. Head to www.dianamatuszak.com/work-with-me/ to download the e-course.

For those who experience this to the point where it affects your quality of life, I suggest looking for outside support. Hire a coach or seek therapy for guidance. It's time to face the beast.

3. Make clear action steps.

Identify new and improved habits that are in line with the version of you that we just imagined in your dream life scenario that you are working to become. When situations arise that normally cause you to choose an unhealthy coping mechanism, what are you going to do instead? Along with this, what are you going to need to do to ensure you are going to follow through with the better response habit? A reminder in your phone? A bracelet or ring that serves as a reminder for the changes you are working hard to make? This is going to take practice and be challenging, which is why I suggest beginning with the smallest one, or the one you will find the easiest to overcome. You've got this. You're stronger than you think.

On the same note, this is why I am such a huge believer in finding balance. When your action steps allow for things like popcorn when you go to the movies, or dessert during your week—making sure nothing is off limits—these sorts of things lose their hold on us. It's no longer a thrill to have it, so we don't feel the need to devour it and go get more. It no longer creates the "happy" feeling it once did when it was on our list of forbidden things. You take away its power in feeding emotion because emotion is no longer a part of it.

You have a healthy lifestyle you stick to and it's just that, a healthy lifestyle. The same goes for cleaning up other areas of life. Make it balanced, one step at a time. If you want a new career, what is the first thing you can do to make it happen? Focus on that, not the other things necessary to complete the goal. Kapeesh?

4. It's not overnight.

As much as you may wish you could just decide you're going to get over this and never ever do the bad habit again, that's just not the way it works. Like anything else, this is a practice and over time it will become easier for you until it's no longer a part of your being. Understand and remind yourself that this is not a linear process. Give yourself grace and forgiveness. Every day, try to be better than the you you were yesterday. The kinder and more compassionate you are toward yourself, the clearer you'll be able to see the direction you're moving in and become the very best version of you today.

5. Track your progress.

When you begin a journaling routine, it allows you to look back and see the progress you have made. When you're consistently focusing on yourself and working to be a better version of the you you were yesterday, it becomes a much less daunting task. Every morning, journal about your perfect day. Journal everything from what you want to accomplish to the feelings you want to be feeling. Every evening, journal about what you're proud of and what you're going to improve tomorrow. I put this into my twenty-one-day lifestyle guide to creating a balanced healthy lifestyle because I believe it has substantial power in actively rewriting your habits. To grab your twenty-one-day lifestyle guide head to my website (www.dianamatuszak.com).

6. Commit to living a freaking awesome life.

It can be intimidating to begin to take action in the areas of your life that are causing you the most sadness or frustration. It feels so much easier to just deal with what you have, hoping it will change or improve on its own, but it won't. You know what they say, "The grass is greener where you water it." I truly believe that triumph comes after the struggle. You have to be willing to get uncomfortable to feel better. Everything is uncomfortable until it isn't anymore. Become a master of facing the hard and doing the things to fix it. Only then will you be able to truly live freely and spend the rest of your life living your best life.

It's time you face what's holding you back from becoming the person you were born to be. It no longer has control over you. You *can* achieve all of those goals without burnout, without ending up in disappointment or overwhelm. You *will* create your best life.

If you or a loved one is struggling in a way that affects your ability to function at work, have normal healthy relationships with friends, or interferes with your mental or physical health, I encourage you to seek help outside of yourself. I want you to know that you're not alone. You deserve to live a truly amazing life. You deserve to be *you*, the very best version of yourself, right now. It's available to you. Asking for help is not admitting weakness, it is showing how strong you truly are.

As you can see, everyone's story is different. Most people are dissatisfied in some area of life and find that using over-consumption or restriction of food is a natural coping mechanism. Regardless of which side of the spectrum you're on during this season of your life, you will not find success in the food itself, but in improving the area that is making you unhappy. Alright, friends, get out there and get to work making that dream version of yourself come alive!

CHAPTER 8

The problem isn't your body, it's what you think of it.

"The more I like me, the less I want to pretend to be other people."

—Jamie Lee Curtis

A LRIGHT, MY FRIENDS. We are about to get real down and dirty with two words that just might make you cringe. You might get a little squirmy in your seat, making the hairs on your arms stand straight, real cute. You just might rather talk about metaphysics or conspiracy theories instead. But by the end of this chapter, you're going to be feeling warm and fuzzy about it and feel like it's your new best friend. As you can see, we've got a lot to look forward to, so let's hop to it, shall we? Those two little words are: body image. Yikes.

Those words are thrown around today so much they've lost their real meaning. For a lot of people, they've turned into a fad. This is both a good thing and a bad thing. It's good because people are finally starting to talk about it and work toward helping others improve their own body image. On the other hand, it's not so good because it's turned into a concept as basic as pumpkin spice lattes on the first day of September. Body image can be ignored, talked about too lightly, and even politicized at times.

I believe in loving your body at every size. I believe in self-love and self-growth. I believe that no certain body type is the cause for happiness or success. I believe that eating well and being intentional about *what* you eat is important. I believe in pushing yourself to create a healthy exercise program. I believe there's nothing wrong with wanting to work toward a stronger, more fit body *when coming from a healthy mindset.* I believe in consistently choosing to do things in line with the highest version of yourself. I believe in unconditional self-love.

Enter, body image. Body image plays a lead role in developing a healthy mindset. It will never be "perfect," everybody has bad days. But when you're strong enough in your sense of self-love, those bad days don't turn into weeks or months. You can find happiness and success can be found in every area of life, *regardless* of what you look like, and you can do this with an amazing relationship with your body.

What is body image? "Body image is how you see yourself

when you look in the mirror or when you picture yourself in your mind. It encompasses:

- What you believe about your own appearance (including your memories, assumptions, and generalizations).

- How you feel about your body, including your height, shape, and weight.

- How you physically experience or feel in your body.

Many people internalize messages starting at a young age that can lead to either positive or negative body image. Having a healthy body image is an important part of mental health[15]."

Body image plays a major part in creating a healthy lifestyle, whether we realize it or not. I did not see the need to focus on improving my body image during my weight loss efforts at first, nor did I see it while struggling with disordered eating. Rather, I thought it was something that would just naturally improve along the way. False. It wasn't until I recognized that body image would be a lead player in my success with creating a healthy lifestyle that I started to pay attention and work on it. And here's the kicker—*only* after working on it did I finally find success in creating a balanced healthy lifestyle.

Growing up in northern Michigan, right on the coast of

15   "Body Image," NEDA, (https://www.nationaleatingdisorders. org/body-image-0).

Lake Michigan, going to the lake in the summer felt like my home. It's the way I wanted to spend every day when I was a child and it was how I wanted to spend every day as an adult too, especially if I didn't have to worry about things like bills, vacuuming, and other duties. My favorite beach was Haserot Beach, at the very end of Old Mission Peninsula, tucked in a little alcove of east bay about twenty minutes north from my home. Going to this beach as an adult represented the carefree life I had lived every summer growing up, and what a saint my mother was, because she took me there almost every day, rain or shine. She truly is a superhero, let me tell you. This beach still brings me feelings of peace, play, contentment, and security.

Summer going into my junior year of college, my mom, sister, and I headed to our favorite beach for the day. I was wearing my new Victoria Secret bathing suit, which I had to buy a size smaller than before because of having lost more weight than I needed, the bottoms sagging off of my caboose. After going for a swim, I came back to my chair, my sister still in the water, when my mom said, "Natalie is worried about you. She thinks you look really thin." Mind you, my sister and I grew up with a sibling rivalry from hell. It was like Cinderella and her evil step-sisters. I was Cinderella, of course. It took until I was about twenty-three for my sister to realize I'm actually a pretty cool human, if I do say so myself. Upon hearing that she was worried about me, I grew concerned. Natalie? Worried about me? Part of myself—the highest version of myself—had known for a while now that I had gone too far. After studying abroad in Greece and realizing that my fear of less-than-nutritious foods had grown out of control, I knew I needed to stop.

Hearing that my sister was worried about me stirred up a mix of emotions. Part of me was scared and concerned for myself, urging myself to get a freakin' grip on my obsession. Another part of me was excited that I'd finally become one of those "skinny" girls. Despite knowing that I needed to find some sort of balance and work harder to be truly healthy, this excited part of me didn't want to stop until the last layer of stomach fat was gone. Every time I looked in the mirror, I'd pinch my belly, willing the pouch to get smaller. I didn't have much muscle because I wasn't eating enough to keep the muscle I had. I remember putting my hand around my arm, finding gratification in almost being able to close my hand, feeling hardly any fat under my skin., or lying down on my side at night to feel my hip bones protrude—the hip bones Nick just loved to see. But no matter what, the only thing I would notice in the mirror was my belly. My eyes resting on the layer of fat still there.

After that day at the beach and despite my desire to keep losing weight, I took a step back and looked at myself. Other people found me so thin, yet I still saw myself as having excess weight. I couldn't see what others saw. I thought, "If she's worried about me, maybe I need to listen to the part of me begging to stop obsessing." I willed myself to listen. I asked God to help me get better.

It took a very long time for me to be able to ignore that little devil on my shoulder, the one who congratulated me every time the number on the scale dropped or noticed how thin I could make my arm look. I knew I wasn't truly happy and I was beginning to realize that even with a much smaller body, happiness, confidence, and all-around better life was not coming. Instead, it was getting further and further away.

It was then that a virtual light switch turned on in my mind. I realized several things. I thought, "If I feel better about my body, then I'll feel better about my confidence." I would feel better about my "progress"—my value, my happiness—and all of the things I had actually wanted improvement in as a side effect of a smaller body. Then, I thought it might be possible to work toward things that actually make me feel confident and like a kick-ass lady.

That was it. I'd had my first taste of improving my body image.

I'd heard people talk about body image before, but I'd never really focused on it. All I cared about was which foods would give you a smaller stomach and those that wouldn't, or which workouts to do to lose more fat. I focused on every little thing to get rid of the fat on my belly (or what was left of it) in hopes of finally feeling good about myself. I was fully convinced that until that came, I would not be able to have a fully positive body image. It can be tricky too. With exercising and eating nutritious foods, you *do* feel really good. But there can also be a major part of you that also knows you've taken it way too far. It's difficult to hear the higher version of yourself when the worst masks itself at times.

Man oh, man, my lanta, how I wish I'd had a role model like myself back then. I needed my twenty-five-year-old self when I was twenty. Looking back on it, I can see that I thought I was "too good" for self-development and self-improvement. "Self-love" sounded like a load of self-centered bitchery that I didn't want to partake in.

WRONGO, Di, said like the Grinch with my index finger waving back and forth. I thought I was above it, as if I was a stronger person than that. My willpower was better than that. That was for woo-woo type of people, and me and woo-woo didn't go together, but I didn't give it a chance. That was for people with no friends, depression, or who were brought up in an unhealthy family environment. I had friends, an amazing family, and all I wanted was a rockin' body. Why would I, Diana Matuszak, achiever of anything I set my mind to, need self-improvement? Looking back, I can see how this was the basis for my thoughts. I didn't want to admit that maybe I did need help. That wasn't in my nature.

Let me tell you that when I decided to partake in this new endeavor, I was astounded. I thought, "Wow, this is really cool and I actually feel a lot happier." So if you are like the old me, well, sister, hear me out. I'm going to break it all down for you. Give you the dirty details of the scandalous truth that applies to every darn human on the planet.

First of all, self-development and self-love are not woo-woo. They are not exclusively reserved for people with serious mountains to climb in their life, though it is a remarkable addition for them. We all need it, no matter where we are at in our lives. You cannot be the healthiest, strongest, fittest, most confident version of yourself if your mind isn't just as strong. You will never see yourself as beautiful or have a positive view of yourself if you do not first strengthen your mindset. While we're at it, give the woo-woo (i.e., manifestation, energy) a chance—it's actually pretty cool. I am now a self-proclaimed "manifesting good vibes" type of gal and I'm proud to say it.

We're so focused on the external appearances while somehow believing that our mental and emotional health will just figure itself out, but that's not how it works. I'd argue that when we work on the internal, the *external* will nearly figure itself out (with a good exercise program and nutrition base, of course).

As I mentioned, "body image" is a trendy phrase today, but it is so important that we don't treat it like a fad. Body image is *the beliefs and ideas a person has about their physical body, and the feelings and emotions that get strung along with it.* It's like a ball and chain relationship, if you will. Having positive body image means looking at the things in the mirror we actually adore, like your flawless skin or bubble butt of an a** and feeling love, appreciation, strength, and other positive emotions. It's looking at the laugh-lines on your face and being thankful for all of the happy memories that created them. It's looking at yourself and seeing the beautiful person that was created to be happy, for a purpose, and more than just a freakin' body, no matter what dress size you wear.

That being said, "Ninety-seven percent of women say they have at least one negative thought about their body image every single day[16]." t doesn't help that a normal conversation at brunch with the girls might go a little something like this:

"You look so good, that color is amazing on you!"—Super nice, you-should-keep-her-around friend.

"Oh, gosh, I feel so fat today. This is the only thing that felt comfortable,"—You and Helga.

What happened to "thank you," or "Thanks, I know It's

---

16 "Survey: 97 percent of women have negative body image," CBS News, (https://www.cbsnews.com/news/survey-97-percent-of-women-have-negative-body-image/).

my new favorite color of clothing." You can be humble without putting yourself down. It's okay to say thank you when someone tells you that you look pretty. It's okay to think you have flawless skin. Feeling like your butt looks great in your jeans does not make you self-centered. Loving your dimples is healthy. Looking at the things you love in the mirror and giving yourself a smile should be normal. Learning that those "I look fat today" thoughts will stop having power over your day if we stop telling ourselves we're fat.

This doesn't mean you have to be 100 percent proud of where you are or never try to improve, no matter what stage you're in. It just means that in every stage or journey you go through, you should talk to yourself as if you're talking to a friend. If we start to do this, we'll teach our friends to do so, we'll teach our sisters and mothers, we'll teach our children and future generations. Then Edna (that sneaky b***h) might not make her way into little third-grader minds like she did with me, letting them know that if their spines don't stick out, it means they're not as pretty.

The way you view yourself affects more than your exercise and eating habits. It shows up uninvited without a bottle of wine in every other area of life too. Relationships aren't as strong, causing insecurity that leads to jealousy, dividing partners and leading them astray from each other. You begin to struggle at work, not believing in yourself when you have a great idea for the company, or believing in yourself to take a leap and start your own business. It can result in not having the self-confidence to start that awesome side hustle to pay for a yearly trip to somewhere where you drink from coconuts on the beach. It causes you to frivolously spend money on fat loss pills, endless meal replacement shakes that you don't need, or purchase clothes that help you hide in your body. It disconnects you from God, or that which is greater, questioning how He'd let you feel this bad about yourself and give you so many struggles.

Instead, you could be in a thriving relationship with Mr. Tall, Dark, and Handsome who brings you pancakes in bed with his shirt off and his hair blowing in the wind—joking, but you *would* get to have a quality relationship that you deserve with someone who respects and loves you unconditionally. You could be speaking up at company meetings, showing how much of a smartypants you are and getting promoted early because of your valuable contributions. You could be exhibiting the confidence to make a kick-ass side hustle empire to go somewhere you drink out of coconuts not once, but twice a year. You could have confidence in your finances, using money wisely with the energy and confidence to go out and make more to live the life you deserve to live. You could be tight as heck with the Big Guy upstairs because you talk to Him on the daily and know He's rooting for you, giving you a prosperous and happy life when you let Him know that you trust Him.

For instance, take my client Erin. Erin realized that losing weight (her prior goal) wasn't just about food and exercise. She told me, "I've realized that being the best version of me all starts with my health. I can't be the positive, outgoing, confident, loving Erin if I'm hating the skin I'm in and not taking care of myself or fueling my body with life giving food. Monday mornings help me reflect on the previous week and plan for the week ahead, so I can start making changes to be that Erin right now."

It's not about restriction, eating less, or willpower. It's about nourishment, celebrating food for everything it does *for* us, and using it to fuel the best version of ourselves. Erin realized she couldn't have an easy time with nutrition without cultivating positive body image and mindset. When the positive body image and mindset were there, she got to show up fully as herself: the positive, outgoing, confident, loving person she truly is.

While we're at it, Erin embodied the idea that a positive relationship with food and body can pour over into every other area of life. In our first session she said she wanted a "better body" because she thought it would help her find a true and authentic romantic relationship. She wanted to live life on her own terms and be her own boss. She wanted to feel confident enough to do all of this and live a life full of adventure and excitement. She wanted drive, tenacity, and a strong belief in herself and her capabilities. A year after working together, Erin continues to nourish her body with whole, nutritious foods. She's shaping her body to be strong and confident in a loving way. She is with a man who treats her like the queen she is. She picked up and moved to a new city to make her side hustle her full-time gig and purchased a wellness franchise to show others how to become the best version of themselves as well. She's trusting God and following His plan for her, no matter how scary. Now *that* is using health and fitness to create your very best life. It's available to you too—are you ready to take it?

Erin did come to me with a goal of losing twenty-five pounds, but in our first session together, we dug deep. I asked her, "What would being twenty-five pounds lighter bring to your life that you don't feel you have right now?" When we continued to go deeper, we found all the things that she truly wanted were the things listed above. I encourage you to do this yourself and you'll find that most of your goals come down to something much bigger than what you look like, relating to your beliefs about yourself and your value. No matter what capacity clients work with me, whether privately like Erin, or through my e-course, challenges, or by reading my blog and newsletters, we *always* lay the foundation of coming from a place of love, self-respect, and being the best version of ourselves—mind, body, and soul. When you work on your relationship with yourself first, it all gets much easier. No, I'm not saying it is easy. I'm saying it can be easier than it is now, and soon it will be your lifestyle.

So, let's start a revolution: a revolution of saying "thank you" when someone compliments you and believing them; a revolution of waking up and being intentional about being your own biggest cheerleader, grateful and thankful for your beautiful body, remembering all of the things you love about yourself. Let's actually *do the work* with podcasts, self-development books, self-love practices, spirituality, and more to strengthen our positive body image muscle. You can't just "decide" to have a positive body image. But you can decide to start doing the things that bring about a positive body image and be intentional about giving yourself a big 'ole hug of appreciation.

At first, you'll probably feel a little wonky and awkward doing the things I'm going to suggest, like a high school boy asking his crush on a date for the first time, but that's okay. The more intentional you get, the more you practice, the more normal you will feel. As with most things, the hardest step is the first one. It's easy to say, "Oh, I'm going to work on this," buy all the books and not actually open the page and put it into practice. You have to take the first step. Do it consistently, no matter how funky you feel and before you know it, you'll be well on your way to not hating yourself anymore.

The magic of this chapter is much less about explaining and much more about the how-to. There is no proven formula to turn body image around, but through my work on myself and with countless clients, this is the system that I've found to be the most effective. But it takes work and you have to be willing to make working on it a priority. Here's what to do:

1. Talk to yourself like someone you love is inside (duh).

When you start to be aware and intentional about the thoughts running the show in your mind, you realize how bad it really is. My favorite thing to ask when people have poor body image and negative self-talk is, "Would you tell your daughter those things?" Take, for instance, these quotes from women in a study done by *Glamour Magazine* in 2011 on negative body image:

- "Fat-ass. Lazy bitch. I hate my thighs. I hate my stomach. I hate my arms."

- "Don't eat that. You could probably use an eating disorder."

- "Your stomach is fat. That is why you are alone."

- "Oh my God, look at her waist and legs! We're the same height. She looks like a model. I look like a lumpy sock."
- "You're obese. All the pretty girls are size 2."
- "I can't imagine anyone wanting to have sex with this."
- "Scrawny and messed up."
- "You're bigger than her. Fatty."
- "Big nose, disgusting skin, bags under eyes, ugly feet, small breasts."
- "Please don't let my size 00 coworker notice this huge gut I've been cultivating."
- "You look like an Oompa-Loompa."
- "Huge legs, fat stomach, not pretty enough to attract anyone, ugly in comparison to others."
- "I look disgusting with my cottage cheese legs and stretch-mark hips. Nasty. No one would want to touch me."
- "I'm ugly. Too skinny. Look sick.[17]"

---

17 Dreisbach, Shaun, "Shocking Body-Image News: 97% of Women Will Be Cruel to Their Bodies Today," Glamour Magazine, (www.glamour.com/story/shocking-body-image-news-97-percent-of-women-will-be-cruel-to-their-bodies-today).

No wonder we don't feel confident in our own skin. We sure as heck wouldn't tell a friend or our daughter these things, so why is it so easy to say these things to ourselves? I'm not sure when we decided (or rather Edna decided) that it was okay to talk to yourself with R-rated language, but let's help her switch that. Trust me, I know this talk all too well—I'm not 100 percent recovered from being my own worst critic, but that's because I'm a human. The difference is, now I can hear the lies and harsh negativity and call myself out. Sometimes I literally think "stop it" in my head, and it brings me back to the reality that talking to myself in that way helps nothing, and in fact, makes it worse.

When you catch yourself about to blow up and critique every little imperfection you see, first things first—recognize your behavior. Imagine you're talking to your daughter. When you notice things about yourself that you're not happy with, it's less about forcing yourself to think they're perfect, and more about empowering yourself to feel beautiful along your journey. Instead of looking at excess weight as "disgusting," look at it as stored potential or energy. Potential energy to give even more effort toward your health and fitness goals, your career, or time with friends.

Furthermore, for every negative thought you have, find a positive thought about yourself. Learn to make positive thoughts more prevalent than the negative thoughts through repetition in this practice. This will come in handy on those days when you're just a human and having a bad day. Have grace, be kind, the bad day will pass.

2. Watch your critical eye.

I bet you're assuming I mean your critical eye of yourself. Well, that too, but that's not what I'm talking about here. Instead, watch how often you play fashion police, or make fun of a stranger, or even a loved one. These thoughts are only breeding more negativity. Have you ever heard of the saying, "When you point a finger at someone else, don't forget the three pointing back at yourself?" How is your judgment a reflection of an insecurity of your own? How is this Helga's way of reminding you that you too are unhappy with yourself in some way? If we're trying to be our own biggest supporter, we sure as heck need to support and be kind to others too. A negative thought is a negative thought. Negativity thrives on duplicating itself, whether it's about yourself or someone else. All around, let's be more like Positive Polly than Negative Nancy.

3. Be in charge of your mind.

If you recall back to Chapter Two, when I introduced the concept of the subconscious mind in the horrible form that is Helga, remember that she is actually the one running the show in your mind, creating beliefs based on your past experiences. As Mahatma Gandhi says, "Your beliefs become your thoughts, your thoughts become your words, your words become your actions, your actions become your habits, your habits become your values, your values become your destiny."

But don't worry, you're not stuck with the load of doo doo that Helga's been feeding you your whole life. You do have the power to change your thoughts, and rather be in charge of your mind. Doing so transforms anxiety, stress, health (mental, emotional, and physical), confidence, patience, and so much more.

Here are some ways in which you can begin to feel in charge of your own mind and thoughts:

- **Meditation:** Meditation is any practice in which you focus your mind on something. It might be focused on the breath, a visual, a word or mantra, or an experience. You can begin with short, even two to five-minute guided meditations. Gradually add time as you get used to the practice. There are numerous apps available with guided meditations for different purposes. For example, meditations exist to support having a good day, waking up, calming before bed, reducing stress, focus for sports, and more. Meditation has helped me and my body image by helping to focus on the things I *want* to be feeling: happy, light, energetic, confident, peaceful. It helps to get you to act in the way you want to feel and notice how close the feelings you actually want to be experiencing are and that your negativity isn't doing you any favors. Instead of waiting for the feeling to come, it allows you to be more proactive about it.

- **Affirmations:** Recall back to Chapter One when I talked all about how I thought affirmations were reserved for the woo-woo type of gal. Well, turns out, I like the way those woo-woo types think. Every single morning, make a habit of journaling affirmations in line with the life you want to have. These can be things you want to feel, do, be, embody, and more. I have found that, especially on days I wake up as Miss Grumpy Gills on the wrong side of the bed, they have the power to change my mood and help me move into a more positive space. Further, recite them any time of day you begin to slide back into Miss Grumpy Gills. Positive body image affirmations could be:

- I am smokin' hot.

- My legs are strong and able.

- I am full of energy, abundance, and I radiate happiness.

- I am the healthiest, most fit I have ever been.

- My hair is fabulous.

- I am one sexy human.

They might feel awkward at first, but when you fully embody and envision the *feelings* you want to be having in association with each affirmation, your mind follows suit and begins to feel those things. It's even a great source of motivation to help you continue to make healthier choices and do positive, self-serving things that turn into habits if done enough.

- **Word board:** I particularly love this one. It's like a vision board, but with words. It's a board with cut-outs or written out words that represent the highest version of yourself. If the highest version of yourself is happy, loving, adventurous, patient, or silly, then you put these words on the board. Put the board somewhere you are most of your day, or even make different ones for different places. This could be one for your room, your office, and your bathroom. When you look at the board it acts as a reminder of the highest version of you and the way you'd feel if you continuously acted as her. Does the highest version of yourself nit-pick every flaw she can see on herself? Probably not. She's loving, compassionate, and patient, or something along these lines. The highest version of yourself does not look at herself with disgust. She sees beauty and opportunity. Use a word board along with your vision board to remain aligned with the highest version of you.

4. Tell yourself those three little words.

This one feels all sorts of weird the first few times, but soon, your mind will be rewired and the habit of finding fault upon waking and looking in the mirror will be a distant memory. Say to yourself "I love you," repeatedly, until you feel it. Another way I love to implement this and take it one step further is by writing "I love you" on a pretty index card and taping it to your mirror, or adding "I love ___ about me" every single morning/night to your gratitude list if you have one (which you should).

5. List it out.

Prove to yourself that you do feel amazing in your own body by writing down when you do. For example, if you go to spin class and feel like a kick-ass lady, write it down. If you get all fancied up in a beautiful dress and you're like "damn girl, I look good!" write it down. Write it all down until your list is so big that you have numerous things to pick from when you're having a bad day to turn it around.

6. Unfollow.

I've said this before and I'll say it again. Social media, television, and magazines all affect us more than we comprehend. What do you watch that encourages negative thought patterns? Who do you follow that consistently causes you to question your healthy lifestyle methods, compare your butt or legs to him or her, or restrict your food intake because they do? If you're following someone who makes you feel like you won't get to the most fit version of yourself unless you count macros and you don't want to count things, unfollow them. If for any reason you are taking in content that causes you to criticize yourself in anyway, toss it, gal. Ain't nobody got room for that.

When you combine these practices and work toward doing them every darn day, no matter how new or weird they feel at first, your mind will begin to follow suit. You'll actually begin to rewire the stories that Helga has made you believe your whole life and turn them into truths and beliefs in line with the beautiful person you are becoming. Do it so much that you no longer have to think about doing it and you begin to form the habit. We're talking at least ninety days. No giving up. You may forget a time or two, but keep on keepin' on my friend. This is how a lifestyle is created. Just as working out becomes a lifestyle where you don't workout because you're *motivated* to, but rather because it's just what you do, it's become a habit in your life. Becoming a Positive Polly beaming sunshine and smiles most of the time can be a lifestyle too. Thinking well about yourself is the key to keeping success and goals within reach. Believe you already are the highest version of yourself, you're just letting her out more and more every day.

Sister. When you do this, you gain a confidence, motivation, and determination to stop settling in your life. You discover the person that you were created to be on this earth and you discover your deep-rooted tenacity to go out and be her. Every single area of life begins to feel more aligned, and you put in the work to make it your reality.

CHAPTER 9

The fastest path
to a kick a ** life
is to just live it

"And then there's the most dangerous risk of all—the risk of spending your life not doing what you want on the bet you can buy yourself the freedom to do it later."

—Randy Komisar

HAVE YOU EVER considered the fact that your health and fitness is actually related to your career? Now, you might be asking yourself, "Does it actually have anything to do with my future and likelihood of success? I mean, seriously. Does getting my Namaste on or picking up a dumbbell and putting it back down repeatedly really impact what pays the bills and my likelihood of chillin' on a yacht in the middle of the French Polynesian coast?"

Yes. Yes, it does. Now, for the grand finale firework finish. I'm going to show you how to take the foundation of your healthiest body and mind—what we've been building together in this book—and use it to catapult you into living the high life. First though, let's uncover what *your* high life looks like. I'm going to show you that you get to live this seemingly fantasy life that doesn't have to be a fantasy at all. It can be real for you. Even creating the kind of happiness and life satisfaction that makes you wake up immediately with the alarm and stretch your arms nice and big, a huge smile on your face like those commercials for sleep aids. You continue your day cheesein' like a little kiddo who just found out she's going to Disney World! Does that sound like fantasyland where unicorns frolic and the sky is always blue? You're right, it totally does, at first glance.

But what if finding happiness in every day, being completely at peace, and feeling like you're doing exactly what you are meant to be doing on this earth was actually true success? What if the Disney-level joy I described above is what it would feel like to live like this day after day, most of the time (not perfection, friends)? Life is meant to be thoroughly enjoyed. Whether adventuring through the Rocky Mountains and knocking Mount Everest off your bucket list is your version of living life to its fullest, or cooking some Martha Stewart-style meals at home and thriving while living the simple life is your definition of success. Either way, you were born to have that. Every human is born with the right to live life to its fullest, in whatever capacity that means to you. You deserve it, you are worthy, you are capable.

The topic of living an epic life is hot right now. So many bada** men and women are working to spread the word that life is meant to be lived NOW, not after years of working yourself into the ground to finally have enough money to "be able to live the life you want."

Here's my take on it. We are all created for a purpose. We all have a blueprint, already prepared by the big man upstairs that is even more juicy and fabulous than we can possibly dream up right now. If we all followed this plan, there would be much more happiness in the world, and less struggle and strife. But over time, Helga and Edna start to convince us this isn't necessarily true. They put on a great act, and before you know it, you no longer believe life can be how you imagined or that it can be even better. Our patterning (our thought processes, default emotions, and way of being) is that of Helga and Edna's lies.

Many of us have grown up and lived in the society where you work to pay the bills, save up enough dough to be able to take those fascinating vacations or buy the dream home when you reach retirement, and *then* start living the blissful life. As if finding fulfillment in your everyday life (mainly your career as it engulfs most of our days) comes second to playing it safe and secure. Leave the high-paying, secure job that works you like a dog, where you feel empty and depleted, to pave your own path? That's irresponsible. Choose a major you're passionate about and enjoy doing over the one that's guaranteed to give you a job the second you graduate? Stupid. That's the mask so many of us have been given to wear. There is a difference between settling for something that's "easy" instead of going for what may be more secure, and doing what you love though less secure, with the drive to put every ounce of effort you have to make your dream a reality. Make sense?

But now, friends, we're starting to wake up. We're seeing the light and beginning to follow the path laid out for us by our maker or the universe instead of the one that a fear-driven society has instilled. The first pre-laid path that is far more magnificent than we ever could have dreamt up on our own. We co-create with God the reality we are meant to have, to not only live a thriving life, but to contribute to the world in the way our greatest strengths are highlighted. We make the world a better place, one thriving person at a time. How amazing that living your best life is the new black?

Throughout this book you've been given numerous tools, exercises, and pattern rewiring techniques to be able to call out Helga and Edna on their misinformation and get to work rewriting those thought patterns and beliefs into what is actually true. You can now gain a level of confidence you've never felt before. You can identify the things you're so gosh darn good at and love doing more than anything. You can discover your strength, what's possible for you in your life and begin to pursue it rather than listen to the "You really think you can do that?" voice in your head. So, back to dumbbells. Specifically, picking them up and laying them down. Foot to pavement, padded cycling shorts to incredibly uncomfortable cycling seat. What does all that have to do with your future, your career, and success?

Finding the courage to identify Helga and Edna's dishonesty, admitting to their current power and influence over you and actively deciding that you're ready to start following through on what's actually true for you, which is not a small beast to tackle. It requires a big ol' dose of putting your big-girl pants on, digging up your inner confidence muscle, and doing the squats of all squats on that confidence muscle to get it as strong as Mr. Arnold Schwarzenegger in the confidence world. Enter: dumbbells, pavement, and padded cycling shorts.

Arguably, the very best part of creating your most balanced healthy lifestyle is much less external and much more internal. The transformation of your mind, your belief in yourself, your determination and drive, your willingness to buckle down until the goal is met, all of these become stronger than we ever imagined they could be once we identify Edna and Helga as the crude con artists of our minds and begin *giving ourselves permission* to be in charge of our own decisions and life path.

Changing your lifestyle for the better is tough. Replacing most of your donuts with protein-packed green smoothies or turning weekend binges into weekend workouts requires more than just relying on motivation every day. The same goes for identifying and pursuing your purpose on this beautiful earth. Recall that when one area of your life improves, the others begin to improve as well, as if by default. But it's not by default, it's because of you. You see, when you begin to stick to the healthier lifestyle you've set out to accomplish, you use that sense of challenge and accomplishment more often in other capacities than in the past. You might push yourself harder in the gym than you ever thought you could, or you might become more intentional or creative with the meals you cook to keep them nutritious yet tasty. *You stick to it no matter how slow the process may feel.* You begin to feel the results of your efforts. Then the magic happens, sister. Then you begin to feel the way you were created to feel. You have endless energy. Your mood is consistently elevated. You understand the memes of people walking out of a workout class like they're America's Next Top Model. You sleep like a baby. You find joy in the little things.

With this, you gain a sense of self-awareness that feels as if you've finally found the real you that's been hiding under all of your insecurities and self-doubt. This is a non-judgmental process. Everyone goes through periods of intense insecurity and self-doubt. You're not a failure, you're human and now you're growing and improving. You're confident in yourself, in your appearance, in your skills, in your strengths, in what you stand for, and in what you stand against. You're aware of what lights you up and what brings you down. Going one massive leap further, you take your awareness and turn it into action. You start saying no to things that bring you down, and yes to more things that lift you up. This includes activities, people, places, jobs, horrifyingly hot yoga classes, and more. You begin to see Edna pop up in places you never knew she was sprinkling her bad juju all over, and you tell her to talk to the hand because the face ain't listenin' to all of her uninvited actions. You no longer let Edna or other people affect your decisions or get under your skin as easily as they could in the past. You form a sense of self-awareness and respect that acts as an armor against everything not meant for you in your life. You learn the difference between what you feel you "should" do and your true desire.

Picture this. We're all just a bunch of confused souls trying to find ultimate happiness while simultaneously trying to pay the bills, trying to find work/life balance and a sense of fulfillment. How many times a day do you say, "I should . . ."? I had a mentor once tell me to stop shoulding all over myself and make a decision. I thought, "Wow, this girl knows what she's talking about." "Should," "could," and "would" are all words that hold us back. They contribute to the conflicting versions of ourselves that never seem to agree with each other.

Let me lay it out for you. We have our "ideal" self, our "actual" self, and our "ought" self. The actual self is who we are today. Not who we "think" we are but who we actually are, including our habits, our personality traits, the decisions we make, and the things we both like and dislike about ourselves. The ideal self is the one where if I were the highest version of myself, freely exuding everything that makes me "me," the very best version of me, this is who I would be. It's the version of yourself that your gut and intuition are working to mold you into. It's a combination of all of your strengths, your passions, your skills, and the things that make you the best person you can be. The "ought" self is who we think we *should* be, or who we think other people want us to be. Also known as, Edna's version of us.

Junior year of college, in the midst of going through massive amounts of self-growth and discovery, getting much closer to my version of a healthy balanced lifestyle, I began to recognize these conflicting versions of myself. My actual self was learning what lights me up and what brings me down. I became even more aware of the fact that consistent partying until the wee hours of the morning and getting drunk was just not something I liked to do on a regular basis. But I was going anyway, because I felt like I *ought* to go in order to be liked. That's what people my age do, right? If I don't, what would people think of me? Would I be rejected? Made fun of? I was in the process of strengthening my confidence muscle, but it wasn't quite there yet. I couldn't just be myself and be confident in my identity. Not yet.

Furthermore, I had a desire to live a life of adventure. Going new places, meeting new people, going out to fun restaurants, doing new things outdoors, everything that makes me as happy as a little kid in a candy store. At that point, I was pursuing a career in accounting and economics. My goal for many years was to move to a big city and intern for a large accounting firm, possibly making that city my new home. Business was rooted in my soul and I wanted to see how far I could go with it. Remember Nick? Of course, how could you forget. Nick didn't want me to do that. Nick wanted me to stay in our hometown, intern for a local firm, and leave that sense of adventure behind.

"You could work for Plante Moran, my co-worker's wife works there she really likes it. Just imagine, you could be at home with the little kiddos, maybe we'll get a dog! A hunting dog I can take with me out onto the farm. We'll be right by both of our families, we'll have plenty of help if we need it. I can't wait," Nick said.

Willing myself to see that as fun, I replied, "Yeah, we'd be by our families, I guess."

For a year, I denied the fact that Nick and I were polar opposites. From an external view, my family thought he was perfect. He treated me well (in front of them—they were unaware of his harsh comments), and they thought we would live a "safe" life together.

Nick would continuously express his dreams of the

two of us settling down out on Old Mission Peninsula, getting married right out of college, and starting a family. Desperately, I tried to convince myself that I, too, wanted that life. Deep down in my gut, my intuition was telling me that was not the life for me. I didn't want to move right back home to the town I spent majority of my life. I didn't want to be a mother right away. Eventually, yes, but not right away. I worked too hard to not even consider having a more thriving, adventurous career. I also didn't want to be with him. We didn't have the same goals, desires, outlook on life, or much else. He was in love with the *idea* of me. A blonde, thin, smart girl to have for arm-candy. Of course, he wanted to make sure I remained the perfect view of that image. Not *the real me*. The stubborn, impatient, compassionate, hard-working, and headstrong me. Regardless of how thin or not thin I was. Regardless of what I looked like at all. I was more of an image to him instead of a person.

Numerous books, podcasts, positive influences, and heartfelt talks with God later, I began to find my confidence, my identity, and my true self. With a good amount of practice, my confidence muscle began to become the strongest it's ever been. I said goodbye to Nick. I found appreciation for my body *regardless* of how it looked. I landed the internship of my dreams in my favorite city, Chicago. I began to mend my relationships with my friends. Day by day, I was finding myself.

Mind you, my "ought" self was still making an appearance. But despite the stubborn power of my "ought " self, I loved my summer in Chicago and I was getting closer to the healthiest version of me, especially mentally. I wasn't there yet, but I could feel the reward of finally getting closer. Each day I was becoming more self-aware, noticing where I let Edna and Helga take over and where I need to knock them down. I enjoyed my job, but deep down there was a part of me that knew my passion for wellness was something special, it wasn't just a hobby. Wellness, nutrition, fitness—they were all my passion. But I didn't "dislike" the career I was currently pursuing, so I continued on. I enjoyed the cutthroat, hard work, and determination it took to "make it" as a CPA, so on I went.

Two years later, I found myself head over heels in love with T, living in Orlando and pursuing a successful career in public accounting. On the outside, I had my s**t together. Nevertheless, that burning passion deep inside knocked on me louder than ever. Wellness was my passion and I finally gave myself permission to see it as my purpose as well.

When you open yourself up to being led by that which is greater and give yourself permission to embrace your purpose and pursue it, your path becomes clear. Within the same week in early January of 2017, I enrolled at the Health Coach Institute where I would pursue a Holistic Health Coach Certification followed by a Masters in the Transformational Coaching Method. During that year, I also joined the Anywhere Office, a community working to change the way the world views health. That is no coincidence, but rather the reward of doing the work and giving myself permission to be the person I was created to be.

I've always been guided to be the best I can be by people who have done *their* own work to be the best version of themselves. For example, I grew up looking up to superdad. My dad created a life for himself and our family that deserves an award. Seriously. He should be speaking to people all over the world telling them the secrets to building a thriving life. Dad's the smartest businessman I know. I was lucky enough to grow up watching him prove to me and our family that regardless of your life circumstances, you can create the life of your dreams. My dad didn't have an easy start by any means. Quite the opposite. He was able to go to college because of the merit scholarship he received—he was not handed success on a silver platter. He's been bankrupt, fearing where he'd find money for groceries, and seemingly hit a very hard rock bottom. He has worked endlessly to give my family an incredible life. His joy comes from seeing us happy. He's one of the most genuinely happy people I know, which is what I love about him most. He's taught me hard work, discipline, and to never give up.

They say girls look for men like their father in a partner. Dad set the bar sky-high, but T reaches it. T, just like my dad, is always happy, has a motivation unlike most people I know, and works his tail off to make his dreams a reality.

T and I have dreams of living a life of adventure, leaving nothing unseen, leaving no experiences behind. We know what we want and we're willing to work for it. Imagine the fear in my mind when I went to tell T that I wanted to quit my very secure, high-paying, steady-progression corporate job. With that job, we'd be nearly guaranteed the income to live that life. But each day I was left depleted, feeling as if there were something missing in my life, like I was not being the person I was created to be. This was until I found holistic health coaching and the Anywhere Office. My intuition nagging at my gut had finally quieted. I knew I was following the life meant for me. T loves *me*. T wants me to be *happy*. T believes in me more than words can explain.

Remember back in Chapter Four when I explained how I told T I wanted to quit my job to be a health coach? His immediate response of "You would be so great at that, when can you start?" was God showing me that T was truly the person for me. It was yet another example that I'd found the one who loved *me*, not an idea of me. He loved my flaws, and my strengths. Not only that, it was a testament to show me that my intuition was finally being heard, and I needed to follow it. The world needs my knowledge, my skills, my compassion, my experience, and my God-given purpose to create more happiness, health, and life in the people around me.

T encouraged me to pursue my dreams, just like my dad had growing up, but I wasn't so sure Dad would be as quick to support my new dream as T. My dad had been thrilled to have me following in his footsteps as a CPA. We'd talk accounting and auditing and I could hear the pride in his voice for me. Tell my dad I want to quit? Tell him I want to be a health coach? Entertain the possibility that he would be disappointed in me? Terrifying. For months, I waited, wanting to do anything but disappoint the person I look up to most.

"Tonight at dinner you need to tell Dad what you want to do. Don't worry, just tell him what you're thinking," Mom said.

In the bar at Shula's in Orlando, my dad's new favorite restaurant, I was shaking.

"Dad, I know you love that I'm a CPA. I really don't want to disappoint you, but you know I've been getting certified as a Holistic Health Coach and I really love it. I can feel in my heart that this is what I'm supposed to be doing in my life. With everything I've gone through growing up and in college, I know God created me to help other people going through what I went through. I want to start my own holistic health coaching business," I said.

"How could I be disappointed in you? That's exactly what I did when I became a CPA. I paved my own path, started my own business. It's tough—it takes years of hard work, but I know you can do that. You have my full support," he said. I had held onto all that fear for months and I didn't need to. He was still proud. It was as if the weight of the world had lifted from my shoulders. Another sign of God knocking me on the head: "Alright Di, is that enough evidence? This is my path for you. Now get to work."

Maybe you're trembling with just the thought about telling people your dream with fear they won't support you. Well, sister, they just might surprise you! If they don't, they're a poop-head and you don't need them anyway.

In the days and weeks immediately following that conversation, I doubled-down on my training, scheduled an appointment with my manager at my firm and said my goodbyes.

Here you might think I'm going to say, "And then everything fell into place and it all worked out!" Oh, Lordy, how I wish that's how it worked. This is what separates those who are successful in the pursuit of their dreams and those who settle for safe and secure. It's not easy. Poop hits the fan, a lot. If you're putting yourself out there as much as you should and giving every ounce of effort you can muster, you get rejected. A lot. Every day, a lot. In the world of entrepreneurship and following your dreams, most things don't work. There is a lot of trial and error. You have to stick with it. You have to be a weird-o, an affirmation-screamer listening to your pump-up jams daily, reminding yourself how to believe in yourself, having high energy all the time, failing, learning, failing again, and keeping going sort of person. Eventually, it will work. You will find what works for you. You'll master it, and then you'll be brought to a new level of poop hitting the fan.

Following your dreams and pursuing the master plan that the Big Guy upstairs created for you isn't going to be all sparkles and dancing unicorns all the time, so why do you even follow it?

When you follow it, every time you fail you will be able to feel God saying "Nope, not that one. Try the next one," and you *still* find fulfillment at the end of the day, even the days you want to pull your hair out. On the outside, a fail looks like failure, but in the world of following your dreams (which are really your purpose), a fail is a win. You're one step closer to finding your unique path to what *does* work. You continue to feel more fulfilled failing on the road to your dreams than "being successful" in an unfulfilling world not meant for you. You're no longer "saving life for later" but rather living life now, in the present, taking advantage of every breath you're given, or at least most of them. Days when you feel like a turd, as if something is "off," will absolutely still come. But with the tools in this book, you now have what you need to let them pass and continue onto your best life.

Stand up more times than you fall down, and you'll be floating on a yacht down the coast of the French Poly-nesian with the satisfaction of making your contribution to the world and having a bank account that reflects your big, fat, juicy role in improving the world with your brilliant gifts if that's what floats your boat, no pun intended.

Now you're thinking, "I thought we were talking about padded cycling shorts and dumbbells as related to career?" YES, SISTER. You nailed it. Paving your co-created path is so similar to paving your way to a balanced healthy lifestyle. Progress is not linear. You fail, you try kale and decide it was the worst decision you've ever made, you head to a new spin class and fall off the bike, you totally crack and forget that you don't go through the hot-light drive-thru at Krispy Kreme anymore. One step at a time though, you find what works. You make homemade kale chips instead and decide healthy can be fun. You head to the bar (as in the squat rack, not the one with tequila) with a trainer and decide the only time you're ever going to look back is to check out your beautiful new booty. You have a delicious cocktail on date night because you're not going all or nothing. You're making balance your lifestyle. You turn your insecurities into strengths, and when you see self-doubt creeping up, holding hands with Edna and Helga, and you decide that you were made for a purpose and continue down the road created for you. Just as working out and eating nutritiously becomes a habit, so does giving your best shot at your goals and dreams. You become resilient, strong, confident, and in love with the person you are becoming inside and out, and you decide that hard work is worth it. You're transformed into the person you know you were created to be.

The transformation of becoming the healthiest, most

confident version of yourself is much more than a new way of eating and exercising, but rather a new way of acting, living, and believing.

So, here's what you're going to do. Ready? Are you sure? Are you really ready? Do you need some water? Alright, great. Now you're ready.

Start living your dream life:

1. Identify your "actual," "ought," and "ideal" selves.

Get nice and comfy with a piece of paper and a pen. Make three columns and label them Actual, Ideal, and Ought.

This is a non-judgmental exercise. It's not about getting angry at yourself, but rather getting curious and identifying all of the opportunities you have to improve. This is a positive action!

Underneath each of the columns, write down words or phrases that identify who you are being or would be in accordance with each category. For example, under my "ought" column I might write "saying yes to someone else when it depletes me instead of finding a compromise." Begin with your "ideal" self. Look back at your past exercises where you got a firm grasp on the person your heart is telling you you were created to be. If you were the very best version of yourself, this is what you would do—how you would act, decisions you'd make, the person you would be. Spare no details! Continue on to the "actual" and the "ought" to identify what is keeping you from pursuing the "ideal" self. Soon, you will begin to feel less guilty, self-criticizing, or insecure pursing your ideal self.

This doesn't stop. As a matter of fact, it *should* be continuously evolving. As we grow as people, our goals and ideals in each area of life—health, relationships, career, money, spirituality continuously evolve as well. A good rule of thumb is to revisit your list every three months or so, and at least every year. Not only will you notice how far you've come, but you'll notice how much clearer and within reach your deepest desires become.

When you're finished, ask yourself how much your current self looks like your "ideal?" What about your "actual" to your "ought?" And your "ought" to your "ideal?" The goal is to have your "actual" (current) self be as close to the "ideal" as possible. This is where Edna storms in and thinks she knows best. Edna is the queen of bringing up the "ought" self absolutely anywhere and everywhere. But you're powerful, you're a doer, you're determined to stop letting her win, and you're creating your dream life, mind, body, and soul, so you're not going to let her ruin things.

To put this exercise into action, what is *one* thing that you can add to your life to get one step closer to your "ideal" self? Notice I did not say, "what is one thing you can take away?" We must consistently focus on the positive to keep our mood and vibration high. Just as with food and exercise, we don't focus on what we "can't have" but rather all of the things we "get to have." We don't focus on what exercise we "have to do" but rather the exercise we "get to do." Pick *one* thing that would bring you just one step closer to the "ideal" version of yourself—not five things, not thirty, not one and a half, but *one*. Master it until it is part of your "actual" self. And then, choose another one. Repeat the process and soon, you will be even closer to evolving into your "ideal" self. Be better than the you you were yesterday and that, my dear, is progress. Remember, this is the powerful work that creates lasting transformation.

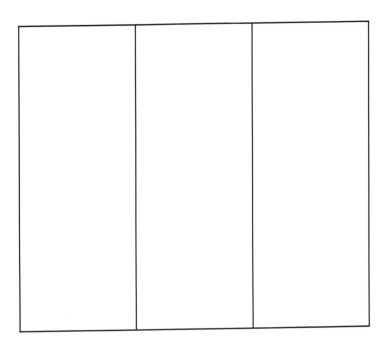

2. Talk it out.

I wish this weren't true, but not everyone is going to be supportive of you. I know that I am one lucky girl with how supportive my family was. I wish everyone could get a reaction like my dad's when they're trembling just to tell the important people in their life their dreams. But in the worst case scenario, there are going to be people who try their darndest to convince you to quit, that you're dumb, and to just give up. Most of the time, this stems from jealousy. I know, I sound like your mother in high school telling you that the mean girl is just jealous of you, but it's true. Have someone else find the courage to pursue a marvelous life and leave them working their mundane job day after day going through the motions living for the weekend? No, they can't admit their admiration for you. Their version of Helga is Queen Bee in their mind.

Instead, talk to those you love. Talk to those you know you can trust. It may not even be friends or family, so find a mentor you can confide in and trust with all your heart. Seek advice, community, mentorship, masterminds, coaching, anything to get you surrounded with other bada** life creating people to support you and your dreams. Discover who will support you and who won't. Decide on boundaries and distances that you need to implement and stick to it. Be open and honest. Talk to God or that which is greater for you. Know that you are being guided.

3. Failing isn't failure, it's feedback.

Tattoo this on your forehead: you will fail. Get that through your head. Whether you're paving your own path as an entrepreneur, going back to school, changing your major, or anything in between, your progress won't be linear. And that's OKAY. Remember, a fail is just notifying you that this option is not yours and to move onto the next one.

4. Affirmations

I don't need to explain this one again, but I hope you now realize you need to write them. Write them as the person you are becoming in "I am" statements and go about your day screaming them through the halls like a mad woman. You've got this, sister.

None of this choosing-your-best-path stuff is easy. It gets tough, but it's the most rewarding and worthwhile struggle you'll ever experience. Except for maybe finally opening that darn jar of almond butter that just won't twist open, ya know? All jokes aside, it's not easy, but the reward is well worth the challenge. Don't be the only thing standing between you and that juicy life the Big Man has planned out for you.

CHAPTER 10

You're a beautiful soul, now go out and thrive

"My mission in life is not merely to survive, but to thrive and to do so with some passion, some compassion, some humor, and some style."

—The one and only Maya Angelou

HOLY GUACAMOLE, MY friends. Oh my, sweet baby Jesus. I just realized I got through giving you so many of my kick a** healthy lifestyle tips and action steps to live your best life and a forgot something MAJOR—earth shattering, ground breaking, I can't believe I forgot this. I just realized this is the first wellness book on God's beautiful earth that didn't mention drinking water. SHOOTSKY. *Facepalm.* So, remember to drink your water, and when you think you've had enough, have some more.

Phew. That was almost so bad. Glad we got that covered.

By now you see and understand that living a healthy lifestyle has more to do with the entirety of your life than simply what you eat and how you exercise, though those are key pieces of course. I hope it's ingrained into your mind, even tattooed on your arm so you don't forget. By creating your most balanced, healthy lifestyle, you give yourself permission and power to create the life of your dreams. Though our focus in this book has been on true wellness, balanced nutrition, healthy exercise, self-love, and positive body image, it was for the purpose of showing you that when you get a grip with these things, your life can truly be what you make it. No longer living by the rules other people create for you (though you should definitely still abide by the law and not be reckless, friends), but instead living the life that you know in your gut you were born to live. The life you were meant to thrive within.

Thrive. Definition of *thrive*

intransitive verb

1: to grow vigorously: FLOURISH

2: to gain in wealth or possessions: PROSPER

3: to progress toward or realize a goal despite or because of circumstances[18]

---

18 Merriam Webster, (https://www.merriam-webster.com/dictionary/thrive).

You were not created to only be sort of happy, pay some bills, contribute a pinch to the world, and then slide six feet under. You were created to thrive—to "grow vigorously" as a human being; to "flourish" into a golden ball of light, radiating happiness, strength, hilariousness, and all of your wonderful traits so bright you glow two miles in every direction; to prosper in a wealth of experience, abundance, and opportunity; to achieve your goals despite crummy circumstances, and power through adversity to realize the dreams that were divinely placed in your heart; to continuously progress into the incredible person you were created to be. The world needs every single one of us for a very specific reason. Regardless of what that reason is, you were born to thrive as that person.

More often than not—because of lousy circumstances such as a hell-bent Helga wiring you into believing you're not special, capable, or worthy, or other atrocious life experiences that make us think we're just not meant to have that dream—so many of us give up. We decide to settle for "good enough." Often times, one, a couple, or all of the different areas of life might set us back, but you were not born to allow those things to keep you from becoming the person you dream to be.

As we approach the end, we're going to go through an exercise I often do with my clients having found this type of exercise during my training at the Health Coach Institute. I find it to be incredibly eye-opening and clarifying when you're not quite sure what's holding you back. It's the concept of living a well-balanced life.

WELL ROUNDED LIFE

Discover what needs to be nourished. Look at each section and place a dot on the line marking how satisfied you are with each area of your life. A dot placed nearer the center of the circle indicates dissatisfaction, while a dot placed toward the outside indicates ultimate happiness.

When you have placed a dot on each of the lines, connect the dots to see your wheel of life. Are there areas where your wheel takes a dive? Are these areas calling to be nourished? How so?

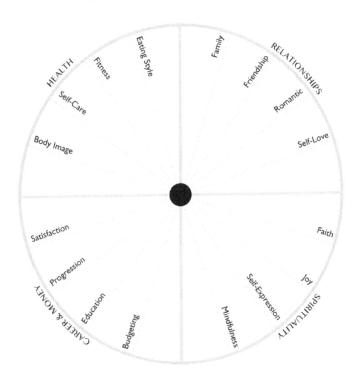

You'll notice that the outside of the diagram identifies each of the major areas of life, with subcategories underneath that contribute to each one. For each of the categories listed above, place a dot on the line according to how satisfied you are in that area. Dots placed on the outside of the circle indicate ultimate satisfaction, and dots closer to the inside of the circle indicate dissatisfaction.

If all dots were placed on the outside indicating ultimate happiness, you would have a perfectly rounded and well-balanced circle, indicating you are living a well-balanced life. Notice where your circle takes a deep dive. Take a minute and answer the following questions:

- What are your top three least satisfied areas?

_____

_____

_____

_____

- What areas of your life are calling for attention and nourishment?

_____

_____

_____

_____

- What areas might be causing you pain, holding you back, or affecting other areas as a byproduct?

_____

_____

_____

_____

- Are some areas lower than you realized?

_____

_____

_____

_____

- How long have you been dissatisfied with that portion of your life?

_____

_____

_____

_____

- Is this something you've ignored, in hopes it might fix itself?

_____

_____

_____

_____

- If you improved your biggest dissatisfaction by just twenty-five percent, what would that do for you? By fifty percent?

_____

_____

_____

_____

- What people, circumstances, or perspectives might be adding to the dissatisfaction in that area?

_____

_____

_____

_____

In contrast, what areas are you most satisfied with? Answer the following questions:

- What are your top three areas?

_____

_____

_____

_____

- Have you always been this satisfied in these areas?

_____

_____

_____

_____

- Do you have an opportunity to recognize how far you have come in a particular area given your hard work?

_____

_____

_____

_____

- What is the primary driver for your success in that area? Can you use this and apply it to your bottom three?

_____

_____

_____

_____

- What people, circumstances, or perspectives have allowed you to experience this success?

_____

_____

_____

_____

Finish with the following questions to turn your awareness into action:

- How might you include more nourishment and attention to your lower areas?

_____

_____

_____

_____

- What specific action steps are you willing to take this week?

_____

_____

_____

_____

- What outside support, accountability, or encouragement is needed?

_____

_____

_____

_____

- If you were to take your bottom three and improve them each by just ten percent, how might that improve your everyday life?

_____

_____

_____

_____

This exercise might be eye-opening, it might be nerve-wrecking, or it might be liberating. Now that you've defined what needs nourishment and improvement, let's get to work making those action steps and turning your ideal life into your reality.

We're going to take this one level deeper. In doing this exercise, did you become even more aware of things that truly bring you joy and happiness? Things that invigorate you and make you excited to seize the day? Things that make you feel calm, at peace, or content? What about things that bring you down? Things you may hate doing? Possibly people, places, habits, or conditions that deplete you and leave you feeling low?

Creating this sense of hyper self-awareness gives you the power to take what you've learned about yourself and begin making boundaries to set yourself up for success. Notice the things you listed as items that deplete you, bring you down, or prevent you from reaching your goals. How can you create a mental or external boundary to prevent that from happening? For example, if you're too busy and don't have enough time to focus on the things that truly matter in your life—how might you delegate or eliminate those circumstances most preventing you from having the time you need? Stick to these boundaries as if your life depends on it, because it does.

To bring this all together, under each of the following areas of life, write down what a 10/10 in terms of satisfaction would look like for you. Fully depict the person you would be at a 10/10. How would you think, speak, believe, act, breathe, eat, heck mow the lawn? The more specific and detailed you are, the more awareness you'll create, and clearer action steps will be.

- Health

_____

_____

_____

_____

- Relationships—romantic and platonic

_____

_____

_____

_____

- Career & Money

_____

_____

_____

_____

- Spirituality

_____

_____

_____

_____

By now you've become a wizard at gaining self-awareness. You know what makes you a beaming ray of sunshine and what turns you into the wicked witch of the west. You know what you desire in life, what your soul-quenching goals and dreams are, and your current stance on your way to achieving those. Let's put these all into action, shall we?

Have you heard the phrase, "The things you are passionate about are not random, they are your purpose," by Fabienne Fredrickson? Looking back on all we just uncovered for you in your life, do you now believe this to be true? Have you been acting as if this is the truth? Maybe you're one heck of a funny gal and you can feel that you're supposed to use this gift of yours, but you're questioning how comedy could possibly be your purpose, or how pursuing comedy could support your lifestyle. Well, sister-friend, comedy puts a smile on other's faces, comedy turns a bad day into a better one, comedy allows you to lose yourself in what is carefree and happy, comedy can change people's lives. Do you work a corporate job that you feel excited about, but you're also really stinkin' lit-up when you make a co-worker laugh? How might you incorporate the two? Possibly begin a weekly office-wide newsletter, start a blog for a side hustle, volunteer at local communities as entertainment, pursue a TV show of your own? Big or small, if there is a knocking at your heart that you've got a gift that not only makes you a happier, more well-rounded, all around better human that helps others as well, that is not random.

Another key factor to be aware of is your mindset. Maybe you've heard it before, but this time you're going to believe it and act on it—everything that happens, big and small, will always be coupled with your frame of mind.

"Negativity and positivity use up the same amount of energy. The difference is one will drain you and the other will fill you up."—Cheryl Strayed

A powerful coaching technique is to look for the positive in every single situation. Let's consider the paradigm, "Everything is an opportunity, even when it doesn't seem like it" (Health Coach Institute HMBA curriculum). Here beholds the power of perspective. Consider the possibility that the soul-crushing, cry-yourself-to sleep-for-weeks, smoke-coming-out-of-your-ears-angry events are all actually happening *for* you, possibly course-correcting you to the path that is truly meant for you rather than the one you think is meant for you. Maybe it even makes you realize how deep your desire to achieve success with that goal is, and you will not let these things stop you. You will find your way.

Your thoughts create your actions, and your actions create your life. Though we are not always in control of circumstances, we are always in control of our reactions in those circumstances. Not to mention you have a whole host of people guiding you, urging you on, whispering sweet nothings into your ear, and rooting for you every step of the way. So many people and forces, in fact, you could form an entire minor league baseball team. Enter stage left, spirituality, God, the Universe, guardian angels, and your people. Let's call it your Baseball Team of Spiritual Support, shall we? That feels right. If you think you're creating this kick-fanny life all by your sweet lonesome, well, no. You are the one that puts in the action, but your Baseball Team of Spiritual Support is the one setting everything in place for you that you have no control over. Faith is the vital ingredient in turning "oh, my lanta, this is genius" ideas into action.

You see that I've referenced God, a higher power, whoever your Big Guy is. Well, folks, faith is critical. Let me tell you why. You are one wonderful, powerful, beautiful being, but you don't have to do this all alone, and in fact, you can't. Trying to do this alone slows you down, limits you, and holds you back from your true capabilities. Doing it alone might be working against what God or the universe has in store for you. When you have faith, you allow Him to place His hand where you need it and give you the gentle push you need to go where you're meant to go. You co-create your life.

Without faith, you are having way too much confidence in yourself to not only be in charge of what *you* do, but be in charge of what everyone around you playing a role in your brilliant master plan does too. Oh, but sister, how FREAKING COOL AND MASSIVELY EMPOWERING IS THAT? You don't have to carry it all alone, *and* you have the fiercest back-up singers in all the land and atmosphere! You see, when following those big dreams and desires that just don't seem to stop knocking at your gut, you get to have a team of spiritual and physical doers helping you find that dream and desire at the very perfect divine time. In the world of ordering a pizza from your phone and directly to your bed, and having Alexa order you toilet paper with same-day shipping after you just realized you ran out of while sitting on the John, we tend to want things immediately. But this juicy master plan of ours is not only epic, it's more epic than we can even fathom at the moment. If your perfect plan has you accepting your Grammy of Success in two years after a well thought out plan, remember that your spiritual baseball team of God or the universe and all your guardian angels may have an even BETTER form of success that happens in two and a half years, or maybe eight years.

Regardless, you must trust that when you tune into your faith, listen to your guides, and take action when they tell you to, you *will* live an even dreamier life than the one we've been laying out in this entire book. It may include all the goals you currently have, and it may include better ones, or even more of them.

The question is, are you willing to hold down your end of the teeter totter? It's all sorts of easy to sit in your comfy chair, doing your newly habituated morning routine, getting so giddy and thankful for what is to come, but then quickly forget about your "doer" muscle as soon as you leave your chair. Identifying the goal, outlining the process, and getting everything in place is the painless part. But when life gives you lemons and then makes them moldy when you try to make lemonade, are you willing to find the nearest trash can and start that lemonade over again?

What separates happy and ideal life-successful people from those who are dreamers and "I can'ters" is the keep on keepin' on muscle. If you fall 7,000 times, you've got to make a commitment to yourself to stand up 7,001. You have to be so remarkably obsessed and committed to yourself and your ideal life that it doesn't matter if a bald eagle comes and breaks through your side door window—you're going to keep on keepin' on. If you don't feel that fired up about your dreams, well, you haven't recognized your true dreams yet. Have faith, trust, (and pixie dust?) in the power of co-creating the very best version of you and the finest life ever with you and your baseball team. Don't just be a dreamer, be a do-er.

Now, friends, having that major league baseball team on your side does not mean it's going to feel as smooth as a baby's tush during your expedition to greatness. We know this, and we know it's going to get tough. During those times of immense growth and expansion with guidance, you're going to get uncomfortable. You have to put your doer pants on and be willing to experience the uncomfortable, fully embrace it, and walk through it until it's no longer uncomfortable, because everything is uncomfortable until it's not, right?

Give yourself permission to live that incredible life, to be that bada** individual, to be as happy, healthy, confident, and peaceful as you deserve to be (which is extremely). Are you giving yourself permission? Excuses come in the form of "I don't have time," "I'm not a priority right now," "I don't have enough money," and everything in between. You have to give yourself permission to see those excuses as Edna and Helga and reframe them into things such as "I have time for what's important," "When I make myself a priority I am a better friend, wife, sister, dog owner," or "I have abundant access to all the money I need," and anything else that puts your mind into "I can absolutely do this" mode.

Say goodbye to your friend, Sir Complains A Lot, and put your imaginary earplugs in whenever your jealous sister tells you how dumb you are. Surround yourself with people who resemble your spiritual baseball team in the flesh. Fill your spare time with podcasts that bring you closer to your goals, workouts that leave you feeling unstoppable, friends who cook you healthy AF meals that leave you feeling better than ever, books that constantly remind you to be in "I can absolutely do this" mode, and close groups of other people putting their doer pants on and co-creating a truly outstanding version of you and the life you get to live.

Here are the basics to achieving all of this, which have been explained in this book:

1. Create your strongest confidence.
2. Find your most balanced healthy lifestyle to help you find that confidence.
3. Set up every area of life to put you down the path to success.
4. Tell Edna and Helga to stop raining on your parade.
5. Love yourself.
6. Believe in yourself.
7. Commit.
8. Have faith.
9. Make. It. Happen.

Understand that you deserve this, you are strong enough, you have all that you need, you are worthy, and you were created for this. You get to thrive. Mic drop, ta ta for now, folks.

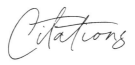

Citations

Intro,
   https://www.dosomething.org/us/facts/11-facts-about-body-image
      (https://www.dosomething.org/us/facts/11-facts-about-body-image).

Chapter 1
   http://www.nydailynews.com/news/national/diets-obsess-tweens-study-article-1.1106653
   https://www.psychologytoday.com/us/articles/200306/our-brains-negative-bias

Chapter 2
   https://wholelifenutrition.net/articles/gluten-free/processed-foods-how-do-they-affect-your-body

Chapter 4
   https://bingeeatingtherapy.com/2011/05/isolation-in-eating-disorders/
   https://www.simplypsychology.org/maslow.html
   https://www.psychologytoday.com/us/blog/the-joint-

adventures-well-educated-couples/201210/women-need-love-and-men-need-respect

Chapter 5 – strength training
   https://medical-dictionary.thefreedictionary.com/strength+training
   https://healthyliving.azcentral.com/acsm-definition-cardiovascular-exercise-18723.html
   http://fitnessorstrength.com/fitness/what-is-liss-cardio/
   https://dailyburn.com/life/fitness/high-intensity-hiit-workout/

Chapter 6
   https://www.healthline.com/nutrition/how-much-protein-per-day

Chapter 7
   https://foodaddictioninstitute.org/what-is-food-addiction/
   https://www.mayoclinic.org/diseases-conditions/binge-eating-disorder/symptoms-causes/syc-20353627

Chatper 8
   https://www.cbsnews.com/news/survey-97-percent-of-women-have-negative-body-image/
   https://www.nationaleatingdisorders.org/body-image-0
   https://www.glamour.com/story/shocking-body-image-news-97-percent-of-women-will-be-cruel-to-their-bodies-today

Chapter 10
   https://www.merriam-webster.com/dictionary/thrive

Made in the USA
Lexington, KY
25 June 2019